The Beginner's Guide to
LOW-FODMAP

Easy Meal Plans, Recipes, and Tips to Calm Your Gut

SARAH MIRKIN, R.D.N.
and the Editors of **Prevention**

CONTENTS

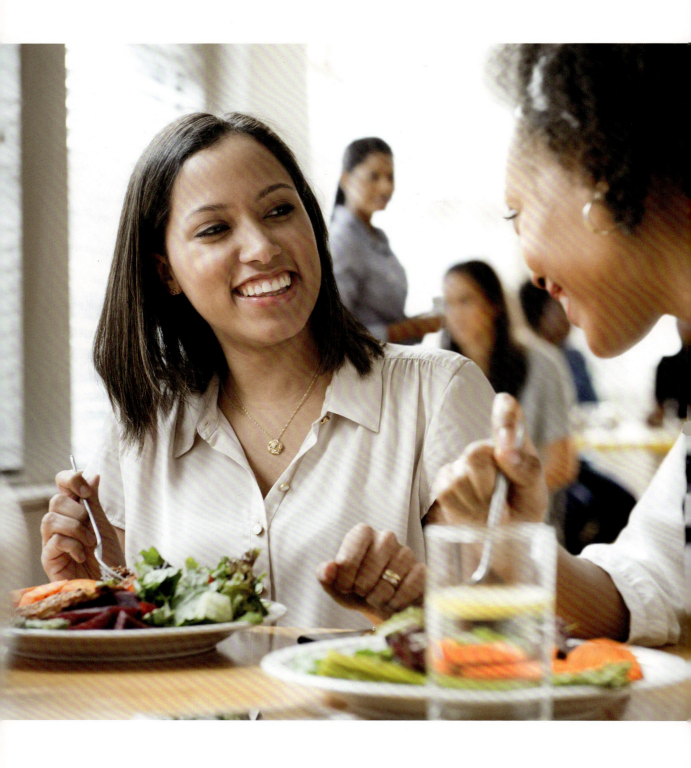

INTRODUCTION: EAT TO FEEL GREAT

Food is supposed to be this great universal: Everybody eats, and mealtimes are the quintessential way of connecting with others. But if you suffer from a gastrointestinal condition, like irritable bowel syndrome (IBS) or small intestinal bacterial overgrowth (SIBO), food can quickly seem like the enemy. You never know what will trigger stomach troubles, and you hardly want to be around anybody when your body rebels.

But what if you could lose the anxiety around food and enjoy it again? Sarah Mirkin, R.D.N., the incredible author of this book, is proof that that's possible. She spent over a decade with a very limited diet because she was afraid to have the bloating and stomach discomfort that so many foods seemed to trigger. There was a time in her life when eating was so challenging that it seemed easier not to eat than deal with stomach pain and discomfort. She says before researchers at Monash University developed the low-FODMAP diet in 2004, finding relief was trial and error. Eating out often triggered anxiety. Even a simple salad could spark digestive discomfort. "I feel like I lost a lot of my younger years because I would have to choose between eating or going out with friends. Sitting at home and having a healthy dinner in my 20's became more appealing than trying to socialize on an empty stomach," she says.

It didn't take long for Mirkin to figure out she had SIBO, but it took her years to discover the foods that worked for her body. She tried everything from a strict high-fiber diet to a 3-week all-liquid meal plan. Nothing worked.

Then she learned about a low-FODMAP diet. The eating plan focused on limiting a certain type of carbohydrates that are difficult to digest. She started the plan and after a few weeks, her symptoms significantly improved. Soon every meal became a cause for celebration, not stress. "The low-FODMAP diet empowered me to have control over my life again and freedom from anxiety about eating," says Mirkin.

Since discovering the diet, Mirkin has spent the last 10 years creating a low-FODMAP lifestyle that is simple, satisfying—and best of all—delicious. "I never feel like I'm deprived or missing out," she says. Now, her SIBO is completely healed and she's able to navigate busy work schedules, social events, and any restaurant menu without worry.

Here, she shares not only her terrific recipes, but her secrets to starting a low-FODMAP diet and calming your digestive woes, and enjoying every part of life to the last bite.

Sarah

Sarah Smith
Content Director, *Prevention* **magazine**

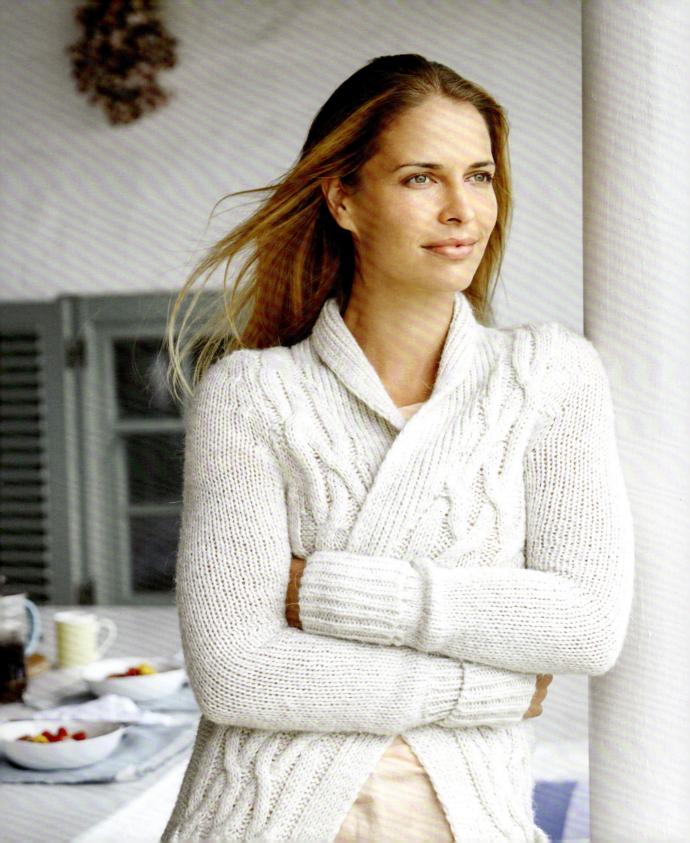

CHAPTER 1

5 Signs Your Stomach Problems Mean Something Bigger

Is there anything more frustrating than feeling stomach discomfort almost all the time? We often assume stomach troubles are caused by unhealthy eating habits: too much sugar, greasy foods, heavy desserts, carbs, or alcohol. In reality, the majority of digestion issues are triggered by something larger than a single junk food binge.

Conditions such as IBS, SIBO, and other gastrointestinal issues can easily be mistaken for "just a stomach ache" but can cause long-term digestive distress. Symptoms can be as subtle as the occasional stomach discomfort and as severe as needing to run to the bathroom at a moment's notice. These issues are characterized by a sensitivity to a certain group of carbohydrates known as FODMAPs (fermentable oligosaccharides, disaccharides, monosaccharides, and polyols). This category of foods gets its name from the process that can occur when these carbohydrates are consumed: fermentation. By the time FODMAPs hit the large intestine, gut bacteria begins to ferment them, leading to gas and discomfort. A healthy gut will break down and absorb food through the wall of the small intestine, but if you're suffering from bacterial overgrowth, food will ferment before it's broken down. This can wreak havoc on your digestion.

FODMAPs affect everyone differently and include everything from garlic to avocado to yogurt. Luckily, with this book's guidance, you can easily manage—and even cure—your GI woes while eating a rich variety of foods. Before you jump in, take a look at these symptoms of common digestive conditions. If you experience any, you may have a GI condition that can be relieved by a low-FODMAP diet. Be sure to consult your physician for a diagnosis and treatment plan.

Signs a Low-FODMAP Diet Could Help

1 | You feel bloated almost all of the time.

Bloating can be caused by a number of triggers. If you get occasional bloating, like after eating too much or having a carb- or salt-heavy meal, it's likely related to water retention. But feeling bloated or puffed up after most meals could be a sign of bacterial overgrowth.

2 | You experience frequent stomach pains.

Normal stomach pains can occur if you suddenly change from a low-fiber diet to a high-fiber diet, you exercise too soon after eating, you eat too many gassy foods, you eat something that has gone bad, or you overindulge. When stomach pains occur frequently and often after eating, it may signal a bigger issue is at play.

3 | Your digestion is rarely regular.

Certain foods are known to spark digestive issues. But if you experience diarrhea and/or constipation regularly, despite a balanced diet, bacterial overgrowth is very likely the culprit!

4 | You're gassy no matter what you eat.

You expect to feel this way after a bowl of chili—but after a typical balanced meal? If you're feeling gassy all the time, it could be caused by bacteria in your gut feeding on FODMAPs. This may produce rumbling noises, discomfort, bloating, and excess flatulence.

5 | You're often anxious.

Anxiety isn't just in your head; it's also in your stomach. Your brain has a direct connection to your gut, and vice versa. The majority of your body's serotonin, the hormone responsible for stabilizing mood, lives in your gut. When your gut is imbalanced, so are your serotonin levels, which can affect anxiety and depression. If you're dealing with anxiety on top of digestion troubles, it might be due to a GI issue.

How can you get relief? By simply altering the foods you eat, you can eliminate bloating, normalize your digestion, calm your stomach, and feel lighter and happier. Read on to learn how to cure your GI troubles once and for all.

The Causes

There is no single root cause of digestive conditions. Some are caused by what you eat. Others can be triggered by medications you take. The cause of IBS is still unknown, but factors such as an imbalance of "good" and "bad" gut bacteria and the aftermath of a severe gut infection may contribute to the condition. The most common cause of SIBO is a bout of food poisoning or acute gastroenteritis. There are many other common causes, including overuse of antibiotics and low stomach acid usually from long-term use of proton-pump inhibitor medications (PPIs). Other less common causes that can be more difficult to treat include nerve damage from poorly controlled diabetes and chronic infection from Lyme disease, among others.

CHAPTER 2

How to Fix Your Stomach Problems for Life

It is possible to undo your digestive problems and still eat a diverse variety of cuisines. After years of cooking with low-FODMAP ingredients, Mirkin has discovered the secret to creating a low-FODMAP diet that is easy, delicious, and sustainable. First, it's important to understand what FODMAPs are and how they can disrupt your digestive process.

What Are FODMAPs?

FODMAP is a not-super-catchy acronym for certain kinds of foods that don't get talked about much: fermentable short-chain carbohydrates (doesn't roll off the tongue either!). On a practical level, you likely won't notice a difference between the six short-chain carbohydrates that define this acronym. Each is distinguished by its molecular makeup and doesn't fit neatly into a certain food group (for example, some dairy products are considered high-FODMAP, while others are not). But if you have a digestive condition, your gut will notice a difference! Here, we break down what each letter stands for.

Fermentable

Oligosaccharides

Disaccharides

Monosaccharides

And

Polyols

Fermentable

Every carbohydrate that's classified as a FODMAP has one thing in common: in some people, instead of being properly digested, these carbs sit in the large intestine and are used as fuel for gut bacteria—a process known as fermentation.

Oligosaccharides

A category of carbohydrates whose molecules are made up of a small number of monosaccharides. This category includes fructans, which consist of short chains of fructose with a glucose on the end, and GOS (galacto-oligosaccharides), which consist of short chains of sucrose and galactose units.
EXAMPLES: wheat, rye, onions, garlic

Disaccharides

A category of sugars whose molecules contain two monosaccharides. There are various types of disaccharides, but lactose is the only high-FODMAP variety. It can be broken down if the enzyme lactase is present. But if you have low levels of lactase (often due to genetics), you may have difficulty digesting lactose.
EXAMPLES: milk, soft cheeses, yogurt

Monosaccharides

A category of sugars that can't be broken down into simpler sugars. There are various types of monosaccharides, but fructose is the only high-FODMAP variety. Fructose doesn't need to be digested, but it can cause problems if it isn't absorbed properly.
EXAMPLES: honey, apples, fresh figs

Polyols

A category of organic compounds that consist of multiple hydroxyl groups. There are various types of polyols but sorbitol and mannitol, which are naturally occurring sugar molecules, are the only high-FODMAP varieties.
EXAMPLES: peaches, celery, sugar alcohols

So what exactly happens when you eat FODMAPs? If you have a digestive disorder, such as IBS or SIBO, you may have trouble digesting foods containing any of the short-chain carbohydrates we just listed. These foods may move very slowly through the small intestine without breaking down, attracting water as they go and triggering bloating. When they reach the large intestine, gut bacteria ferments the FODMAPs, releasing gas in the process. The results? Even more bloating and the potential for other symptoms, including flatulence, constipation, abdominal pain, and diarrhea, depending on your tolerance level. It usually takes at least four hours after consuming a FODMAP for these side effects to occur.

All foods can be categorized as either high-FODMAP, low-FODMAP, or no-FODMAP. Just because a food contains FODMAPs doesn't mean you need to eliminate it from your diet (more on that later!).

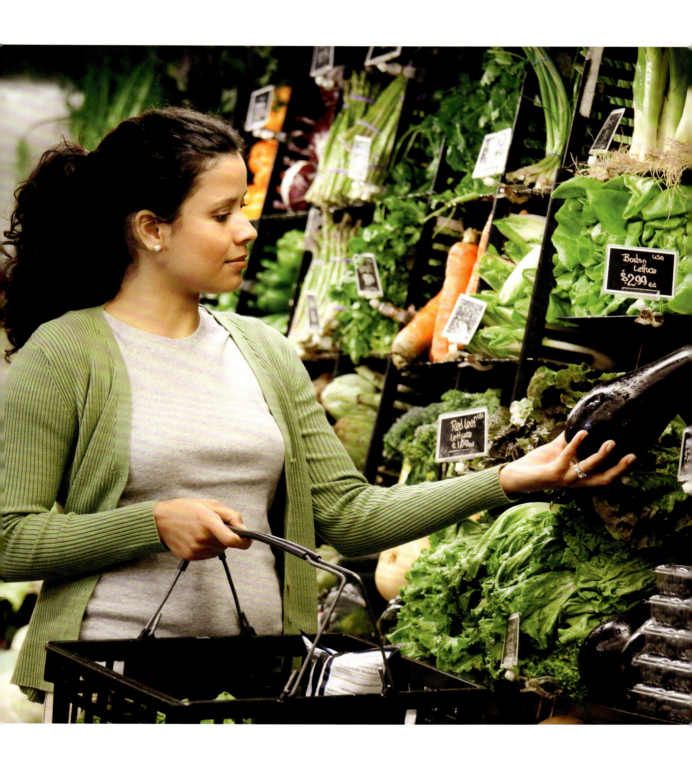

Benefits of a Low-FODMAP Diet

Since it was first discovered, the low-FODMAP diet has helped countless individuals heal their digestion issues. The diet was shown to significantly reduce abdominal pain and bloating in IBS patients, according to 2017 meta-analysis published in *Nutrients*. When you adopt a low-FODMAP diet, you may start feeling relief in as little as 2 days, though it can take up to 2 weeks. That's because the plan is structured to flush built-up FODMAPs out of your system and immediately work to rebalance your gut.

This nourishing way of eating has given dozens of Mirkin's clients fast relief, returning their digestive systems to a level of calm they hadn't experienced in years. One client, Kelsey, who had been suffering from SIBO for nearly 2 years, was able to significantly improve her symptoms, lose weight, and clear her skin. "My mood has also been much happier!" she says. "I'm really well now!" Here's how it can help change your life, too:

Relief from a Range of Digestive Conditions

Low-FODMAP diets have been shown to help people with all types and degrees of digestive issues. Studies suggest that the plan can help provide relief from SIBO, IBS, indigestion, colitis, Crohn's disease, diverticulosis, functional dyspepsia, and gastroesophageal reflux disease (GERD).

Clearer Skin

Studies show that there is a direct connection between acne and digestion. When your digestion is out of whack, your skin acts as an external signal. Many of Mirkin's clients have reported clearer skin upon starting a low-FODMAP diet.

Increased Energy

When your digestion is disrupted, your energy levels can plummet. Fatigue is a common side effect of IBS, according to studies. One *Gastroenterology* study found that when patients' SIBO symptoms were cured, they also experienced increased energy. By rebalancing your gut and curing your digestive condition, this lifestyle can boost your energy levels.

Decreased Anxiety

Studies have shown that digestion conditions such as IBS may be linked to higher levels of anxiety and other psychiatric disorders. By rebalancing your gut, a low-FODMAP diet can provide relief from chronic stomach problems and the anxiety that they trigger.

Weight Loss

When you follow a low-FODMAP meal plan—like the one Mirkin created—filled with a variety of whole, nutritious foods, you may lose some weight because you are omitting processed foods from your diet. However, if you have SIBO or irritable bowel syndrome with diarrhea (IBS-D), you may be underweight and looking to increase to a healthy weight. Because a FODMAP-restrictive diet helps reduce digestive pain, it may encourage those with these conditions to eat more and achieve a healthy weight.

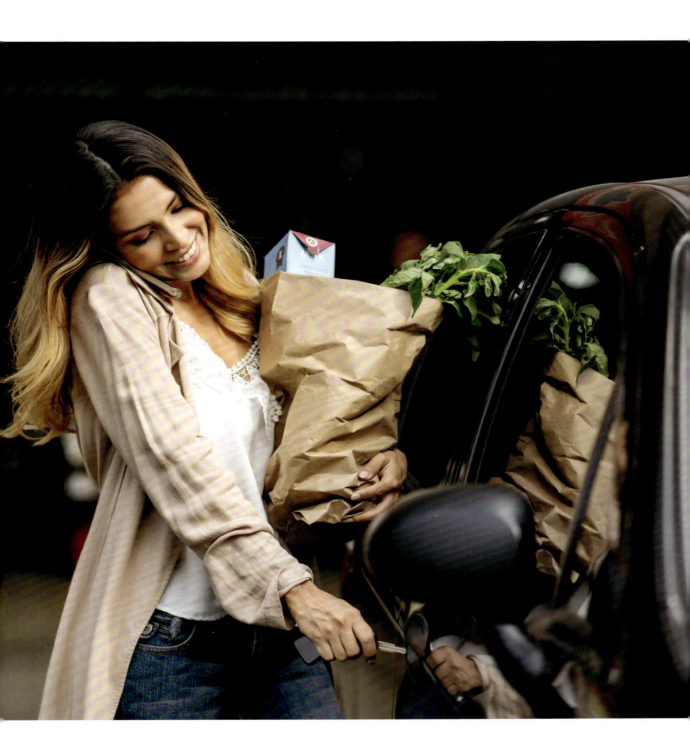

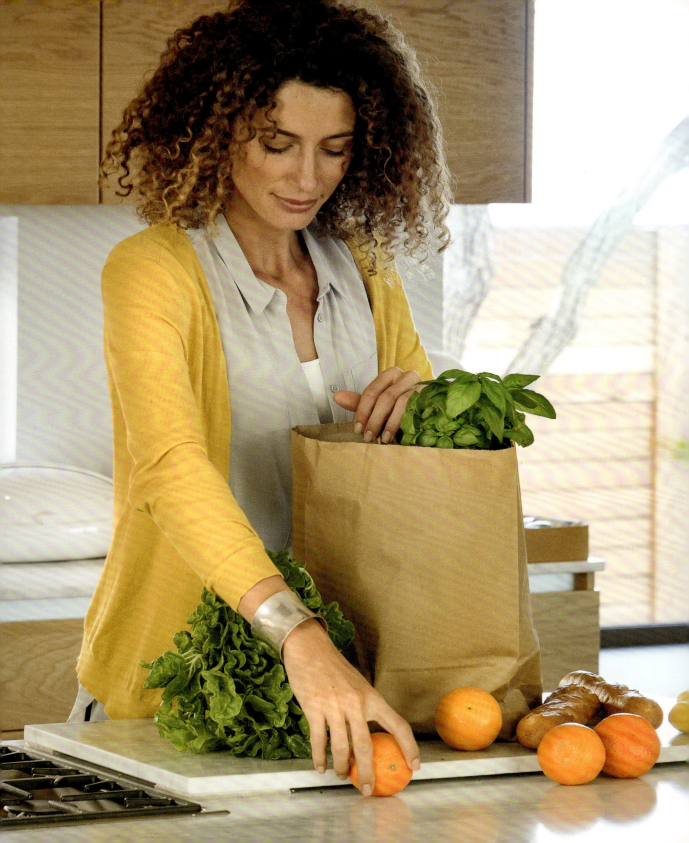

CHAPTER 3

How It **Works**

A low-FODMAP diet works to relieve digestive issues using three tactics:

1 | Eliminating FODMAP foods to flush built-up bacteria and undigested food from your gut
2 | Reintroducing FODMAP foods to determine which you can handle
3 | Personalizing your diet to include the foods that work in harmony with your body

If you follow the plan strictly, your symptoms should disappear within 2 to 4 weeks. Unlike other methods, the low-FODMAP diet doesn't rely on pills or special treatments. Instead, this plan allows your body to heal itself. Mirkin created each day to focus strictly on feeling great, not on counting calories. If your goal is weight gain or loss, it is important to heal your gut first. Here's how that works during each phase of the process:

Elimination Phase

HOW LONG: 3–6 weeks
WHAT IT DOES: Cleanses your gut of built-up FODMAPs
HOW TO DO IT: To start, you'll flush all the FODMAPs and bacteria that may have accumulated in your gut over the course of months or years. You'll begin to notice you feel lighter almost immediately. Once you restrict all FODMAPs from your diet, your body will naturally get rid of what's built up. This will set you up with a completely clean slate for the next phase.

Reintroduction Phase

HOW LONG: 8–12 weeks
WHAT IT DOES: Helps you identify exactly which FODMAPs you can tolerate
HOW TO DO IT: Once your gut is virtually free of all FODMAPs, you can easily discover those you can safely eat and those that trigger a reaction. To do so, you alternate between days that incorporate a single FODMAP into your diet and days that are low-FODMAP.

Personalization Phase

HOW LONG: Indefinitely

WHAT IT DOES: Heals your gut and ensures you live symptom-free for life

HOW TO DO IT: By this point, you've identified the foods that nourish your body and the foods that send it into distress. Now, you can personalize your meals to fit your tastes and your life. Get creative, have fun, and find what you love!

3 Hours

That's how long you should wait between eating the highest tolerable serving of low-FODMAP foods from the same family to avoid stomach troubles.

FODMAP Stacking: What You Need to Know

At every phase of this plan it is very important to note: it is possible for your body to perceive low-FODMAP foods as high-FODMAP if they are eaten in large quantities or within a short time period of each other. This is known as *FODMAP stacking*. For example, ½ cup of canned artichoke hearts is low-FODMAP from the fructose family. More than ½ cup is not. Half a spear of asparagus is low-FODMAP from the fructose family. More is not. That's because the amount of fructose contained in each of these servings is small enough not to trigger symptoms. Eating more than ½ cup of canned artichoke hearts or more than half a spear of asparagus at a time increases the total amount of fructose in your system, which may trigger symptoms. So, what if you consume ½ cup canned artichoke hearts and ½ asparagus spear in one meal? That's FODMAP stacking. Together they are medium- or high-FODMAP because of the combined fructose content and will cause digestive issues. Refer to the complete list of FODMAPs on page 19 for the highest tolerable serving you may have of each during this phase.

5 Things to Do Before Starting

Maybe you've heard about the low-FODMAP diet before but weren't quite ready to start. Follow Mirkin's tips for making the switch totally seamless. Mirkin also suggests downloading the Monash University FODMAP Diet app to help you track FODMAPs when you're on the go.

1 | Go in With the Right Mindset

Remember that starting this diet isn't just about solving your digestive problems. "Think about eating to feel good," says Mirkin. "How much better is your life going to be if you're not constantly concerned about what's going on in your gut?" You deserve to live without anxiety about unpredictable digestion.

2 | Start When Your Schedule Is Calm

You may want to avoid starting the low-FODMAP diet during the holidays, a vacation, or any environment in which you can't control what you eat. You'll have an easier time getting used to your new eating guidelines when you are able to make every meal yourself.

3 | Clean Out Your Kitchen

Remove any high-FODMAP foods from your pantry. Not only will this prevent you from accidentally eating no-go foods, it will also help familiarize you with reading nutrition labels and identifying what makes a food high-FODMAP.

4 | Tell a Friend

Ask your friends and family for support. Let them know that you suffer from digestive issues and how hard you are working to heal your gut. You'll have someone else helping you stay on track and giving you the encouragement you need.

5 | Find Your Favorite Substitutions

Almost any recipe can be modified to be low-FODMAP, says Mirkin. Check out the list of easy low-FODMAP swaps [on the following page] to find delicious alternatives that will keep you from missing high-FODMAP foods.

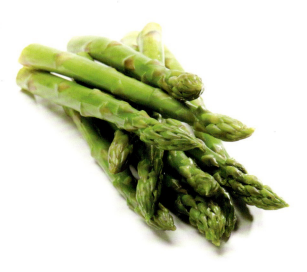

Low-FODMAP Swaps for High-FODMAP Foods

HIGH-FODMAP FOOD	LOW-FODMAP ALTERNATIVE(S)
Agave, honey, or molasses	Maple syrup, sugar
Bananas	Unripe bananas
Beans	Canned lentils, ¼ cup canned chickpeas
Blackberries	Raspberries, strawberries, ¼ cup blueberries
Bread crumbs	Panko bread crumbs, cornflake crumbs, gluten-free bread crumbs
Cashews	Macadamia nuts
Cauliflower	¾ cup broccoli
Couscous	Quinoa
Garlic	Garlic-infused oil
Grapefruit	Oranges, pineapple
Milk chocolate	Dark chocolate (85% cocoa or higher)
Milk or yogurt	Lactose-free milk or yogurt
Onions	Scallion tips, shallot-infused oil, chives, asafoetida
Peaches	Kiwis
Rum	Vodka
Semolina pasta	Chickpea pasta, gluten-free pasta, spaghetti squash, risotto, soba noodles
Silken tofu	Firm tofu, seitan, tempeh
Watermelon	1 cup cantaloupe
Wheat bread	Gluten-free bread, 100% spelt sourdough bread, corn tortillas, brown rice tortillas
Zucchini	½ cup chayote

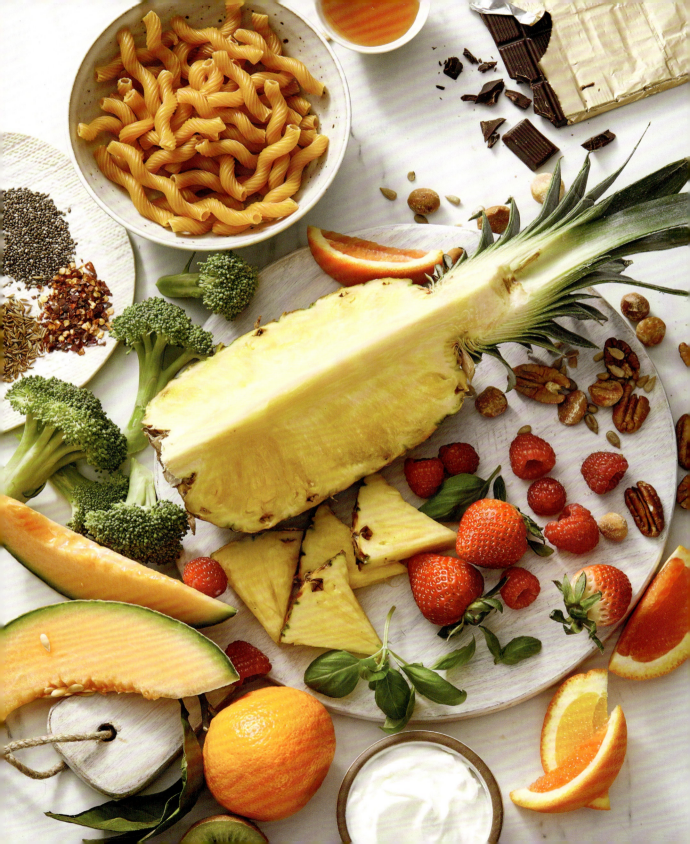

How to Tell If Something Is High-FODMAP

Unlike total calories or grams of sugar, FODMAPs are not listed on nutrition labels, making it difficult to know exactly what products are high-FODMAP. Luckily, if a food has 0 g carbohydrates, you can be pretty sure it's low-FODMAP. Check out the lists starting on page 19 to see which foods are low-FODMAP, which are tolerated in small portions, and which to eliminate entirely.

Here's a list of sneaky high-FODMAP ingredients you'll often find in processed foods and even in medications or supplements. If you see any of these ingredients on a label, it is likely high-FODMAP and should be avoided during the elimination phase:

Agave syrup
Barley
Chicory/chicory root extract/
    chicory root powder
Crystalline fructose
Dried fruit
Erythritol
Fructans
Fructooligosaccharide (FOS)
Fructose
Fruit juice
Fruit juice concentrate
    (e.g., apple/pear juice
    concentrates)
Fruit sugar
Garlic/garlic salt/garlic powder/
    garlic extract
High-fructose corn syrup
Honey
Inulin (sometimes added as
    a fiber/prebiotic)
Isomalt
Mannitol
Onion/onion salt/onion powder/
    onion extract
Polyols
Prune juice
Rye
Sorbitol
Wheat
Xylitol

Make It Your Own: Garlic-Infused Oil

Today, there are more low-FODMAP options in grocery stores than ever before. Mirkin loves FODY brand infused oils, which are flavorful and guaranteed low-FODMAP. But if your grocer doesn't stock them, you can easily make your own. Try Mirkin's favorite recipe for garlic-infused oil:

In a medium saucepan, heat 2 cups extra virgin olive oil on low until oil is warm to the touch. Remove pot from heat and add 6 garlic cloves or shallots. Let sit for 2 hours. Then, into a jar or container with an air-tight lid, strain oil with a fine-wire strainer lined with cheesecloth. Store in refrigerator and use within 3 to 4 days, or freeze indefinitely!

If any of these ingredients are listed on a packaged good's nutrition label—even if it's the last ingredient listed—avoid it. Mirkin says it's better to be safe than risk upsetting your stomach and having to restart the elimination phase.

What to do when . . .

There is a lot to remember with a low-FODMAP diet. Follow these tips for handling whatever comes your way.

You slip up

It can be easy to accidentally eat something high-FODMAP or eat too large a serving of something low-FODMAP, which can have the same effect as eating a high-FODMAP food. If you do consume something high-FODMAP during the elimination phase, you should restart the phase from the beginning in order to fully cleanse your system of FODMAPs and start the reintroduction phase on the right foot.

You're dining out

If possible, review the menu beforehand and identify which options are low-FODMAP or can be easily modified. It can be tough to tell if a food, like plain grilled chicken, has been marinated with onion or garlic. Tell your server you are avoiding onion and garlic, which are difficult to eat around and are so easily hidden in sauces or marinades. If you don't, there is a good chance you'll end up with a dish that has FODMAPs and your efforts will be sabotaged! A good bet? Meat or seafood with a low-FODMAP vegetable or salad greens, and a potato or rice.

The Deal with Dairy

You can enjoy dairy products and still keep your stomach happy! Lactose, the FODMAP found in dairy, is a sugar. If a dairy product's nutrition label has 1 g or fewer sugar, it's virtually lactose-free, says Mirkin. All hard cheeses are low-FODMAP. Soft cheeses, such as cottage cheese, ricotta cheese, haloumi, cream cheese, and sour cream, are only low-FODMAP if you cap your serving at 2 Tbsp.

TIP
If you decide to eat more than 2 Tbsp of soft cheeses, you can take a supplement to help your body break down the lactose, such as Lactaid. Just be sure to check the supplement's label to make sure it doesn't contain sorbitol or mannitol.

CHAPTER 4

The **Elimination** Phase

Now that you know what FODMAPs are, how they can mess with your digestion, and ways to handle a low-FODMAP diet, you're ready to begin the elimination phase. During this phase you must avoid all high-FODMAP foods. If you do this, your digestive symptoms should disappear within 2 to 4 weeks. If you still experience symptoms after 4 weeks, it may be wise to connect with a dietitian, who can help you identify if you've been eating high-FODMAP foods. If high-FODMAP foods are not the problem, visit a gastroenterologist. It could be a sign of a different condition.

It is very important that you avoid high amounts of FODMAPs during the elimination phase. This will allow your body to flush all FODMAPs from your system and set you up for success during the reintroduction phase. Luckily, you don't need to worry too much about checking labels and serving sizes if you follow Mirkin's low-FODMAP meal plan, starting on page 26 in this chapter. She designed every day to include a wide variety of delicious, nourishing foods that will keep you low-FODMAP and keep your stomach happy.

For best results, Mirkin recommends sticking to the meal plan as laid out. But should you want to adjust the plan for weight gain or loss, or add in foods that suit your unique tastes, you can follow her recommendations for adapting the plan on the following pages.

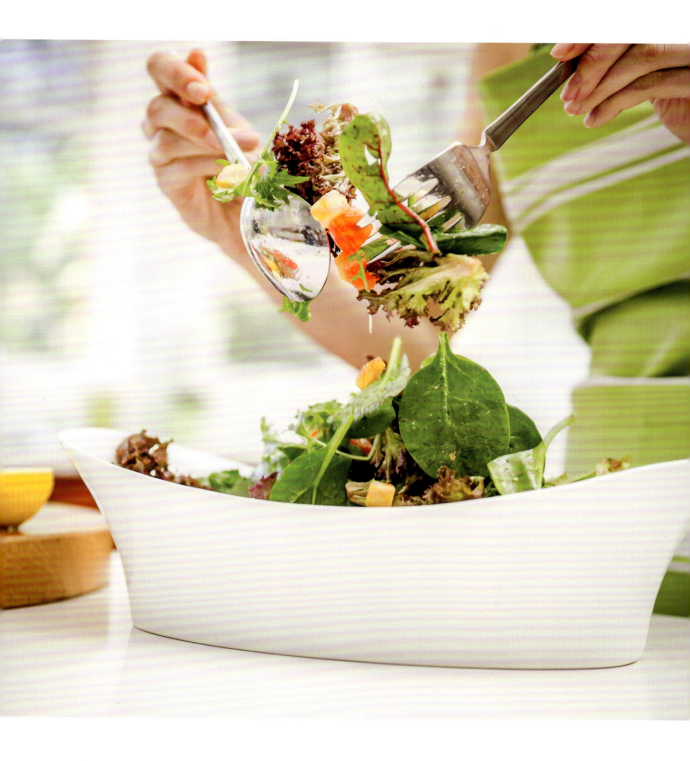

Adjusting the Plan for Weight Loss or Gain

Follow the plan as is to maintain your current weight. If you'd like to gain or lose weight, make the following adjustments.

To Gain Weight

1 | Increase the portion of healthy fats, including oils, olives, salad dressing, peanut and sunflower seed butter, pecans, and walnuts as well as chia, pumpkin, sunflower seeds, and any other nuts and seeds that are unlimited on the low-FODMAP diet.

2 | Increase protein portions, including lactose-free dairy, eggs, and all fish, seafood, and meats.

3 | Include strength training in your exercise routine.

To Lose Weight

1 | Pay close attention to your hunger and satiety cues. Eat when you feel hungry and stop when you feel satisfied.

2 | Keep the protein high in your meals and snacks.

3 | Consider swapping a tortilla or bread for lettuce leaves.

4 | Consider decreasing the portion of some of the added fats in your meals, such as oils, avocado, nuts, seeds, egg yolks, and cheese.

5 | Be a body in motion! Exercise is so important for healthy digestion and feeling your best. Try to include at least one 20-minute workout on most days outside of your regular activity.

Adjusting the Plan for Your Tastes

If you decide to eat outside of Mirkin's recommended meal plan, use the next few pages to guide what you can eat and how much. We've rounded up some common foods and noted which are not tolerated, tolerated in limited amounts, and tolerated at all amounts. Here's an overview of what each category means:

Not Tolerated

These foods contain high amounts of FODMAPs, even in small servings. During the elimination phase, avoid these. During the personalization phase, avoid those that you are sensitive to.

Tolerated in Limited Amounts

These foods contain moderate amounts of FODMAPs. During the elimination phase, enjoy these in portions equal to or less than the amounts noted in the chart. During the personalization phase, enjoy those you are sensitive to in limited quantities and those you can tolerate in nearly unlimited quantities. Be sure to check your intake of other FODMAPs in each category to avoid FODMAP stacking.

Tolerated at All Amounts

These foods contain little to no FODMAPs. During the elimination and personalization phases, enjoy these in nearly unlimited quantities.

Elimination Phase Chart

NOT TOLERATED

GRAINS

FRUCTANS

Rye bread (also high in: fructose, GOS)

Pumpernickel bread

Wheat cous cous

Whole wheat flour (also high in: GOS)

Amaranth flour (also high in: GOS)

Barley flour (also high in: GOS)

Coconut flour (also high in: fructose, sorbitol)

Rye flour

Spelt flour (also high in: GOS)

Freekah (also high in: GOS)

Muesli (also high in: GOS)

Gnocchi, wheat

Wheat bran pellets (also high in: GOS)

Wheat germ, raw (also high in: GOS)

FRUCTOSE

100% whole-wheat bread (also high in: fructans)

VEGETABLES

FRUCTANS

Garlic

Leek, bulb

Shallots

White onion

GOS

Green peas, frozen

MANNITOL

Cauliflower

FRUCTOSE

Dried chipotle chili

FRUITS

FRUCTANS

Dried Mango

SORBITOL

Prunes (also high in: fructans)

Clingstone peaches (also high in: mannitol)

LEGUMES, PULSES, NUTS, AND SEEDS

GOS

Red kidney beans (also high in: fructans)

Navy beans (also high in: fructans)

Pistachios (also high in: fructans)

Soy protein, textured (also high in: fructans)

Split peas (also high in: fructans)

Tofu, silken (also high in: fructans)

Cashews

Semolina

FRUCTOSE

Fava beans

Broad beans

CONDIMENTS, HERBS, SPICES, ETC.

GOS

Hummus (also high in: fructans)

FRUCTANS

Tzatziki

BEVERAGES

FRUCTOSE

Rum

Apple juice

Orange juice

FRUCTANS

Chamomile tea

Herbal tea

Fennel tea

Elimination Phase Chart

TOLERATED IN LIMITED AMOUNTS

The foods below are high in FODMAPs when eaten in portions larger than the amounts indicated.

GRAINS

FRUCTANS

Barley, pearl (also high in: GOS)	⅛ cup
Wheat bran, processed and unprocessed	½ Tbsp
White bread	1 slice
Pasta, wheat	½ cup, cooked
Sprouted pearl barley	½ cup
Gluten-free bread	2 slices
Millet bread	2 slices
Oat bran, unprocessed (also high in: GOS)	2 Tbsp
Rolled oats (also high in: GOS)	½ cup
Gluten-free pasta	1 cup, cooked
Quinoa, white (also high in: GOS)	1 cup, cooked
Corn bread	1 slice
Sourdough bread	2 slices

FRUCTOSE

Sprouted multigrain bread	1 slice

VEGETABLES

FRUCTANS

Pickled artichoke	2 tsp
Beets (also high in: GOS)	2 thin slices
Brussels sprouts	2 sprouts
Artichoke, globe	.53 ounces
Snow peas (also high in: mannitol)	5 pods
Savoy cabbage	½ cup
Edamame, frozen	½ cup
Okra	7½ pods
Red cabbage	¾ cup
Baby spinach	2 cups
Zucchini	⅓ cup

FRUCTANS (CONT.)

Jicama	½ cup
Spaghetti squash (also high in: GOS)	2 cups
Red chili	1 pepper
Broccolini stalks	1 cup
Broccoli	2½ cups
Corn, canned	1½ tsp

GOS

Radicchio	6 cups
Butternut squash (also high in: mannitol)	½ cup
Green peas, canned	¼ cup

MANNITOL

Dulse flakes	2 tsp
Portobello mushrooms	⅛ mushroom
Sauerkraut	1 Tbsp
Celery	¼ stalk
Chicory leaves	½ cup
Sweet potato	½ cup
Leek leaves	⅔ cup

SORBITOL

Sweet corn	½ cob
Bok choy	1 small
Green pepper	½ cup
Green beans	20 beans
Eggplant	1 cup
Fennel leaves	½ cup
Cabbage	¾ cup

TOLERATED IN LIMITED AMOUNTS

The foods below are high in FODMAPs when eaten in portions larger than the amounts indicated.

VEGETABLES (CONT.)

FRUCTOSE

Asparagus	½ spear
Broccoli, stalks	⅓ cup
Alfalfa	2 cups
Broccoli, heads	2 cups
Tomato, canned	¾ cup
Artichoke hearts, canned	½ cup
Broccolini heads	½ cup

FRUITS

FRUCTANS

Raisins	1 Tbsp
Goji berries	3 tsp
Dried figs	⅔ fig
Dates	⅓ date
Currants	1 Tbsp
Dried cranberries	1 Tbsp
Bananas, ripe	⅓ banana
Grapefruit	⅓ cup
Persimmons	½ persimmon
Banana chips	15 chips
Cantaloupe	1 cup
Blueberries	¼ cup
Honeydew melon	½ cup
Kiwi	2 small kiwis
Passionfruits	2 passionfruits
Lime juice	1 cup
Lemon juice	½ cup
Pineapple	1 cup
Raspberries	30 berries
Bananas, unripe	1 medium banana

FRUITS (CONT.)

SORBITOL

White peaches	1½ Tbsp
Apricots	1 Tbsp
Blackberries	1 berry
Lychee	3 lychees
Nectarine	1 Tbsp
Plums	1 tsp
Apple	1 Tbsp
Yellow peaches	⅕ cup
Avocado	2 Tbsp
Coconut	⅔ cup
Shredded coconut	½ cup

FRUCTOSE

Fresh figs	1 tsp
Cherries	2 cherries
Guava, unripe	2 tsp
Pear (also high in: sorbitol)	1 tsp
Watermelon	1½ Tbsp
Boysenberry	5 berries

Elimination Phase Chart

TOLERATED IN LIMITED AMOUNTS

The foods below are high in FODMAPs when eaten in portions larger than the amounts indicated.

DAIRY

LACTOSE

Buttermilk	1 Tbsp
Goat cheese	1 Tbsp
Kefir	1 Tbsp
Cow milk	1 Tbsp
Goat milk	1¼ Tbsp
Goat yogurt	⅕ cup
Regular yogurt	1 Tbsp
Ice cream, vanilla, no corn syrup	⅔ scoop
Sour cream	2 Tbsp
Cream cheese	2 Tbsp
Ricotta cheese	2 Tbsp
Queso fresco	2 slices
Quark cheese	2 Tbsp
Soy cheese	2 slices
Whipped cream	½ cup
Haloumi cheese	2 slices
Cottage cheese	2 Tbsp

LEGUMES, PULSES, NUTS, AND SEEDS

GOS

Lentils, canned and drained (also high in: fructans)	½ cup
Black beans, canned (also high in: fructans)	⅛ cup
Pinto beans, canned	1½ Tbsp
Flaxseeds	1 Tbsp
Almonds	10 nuts
Chickpeas, canned	¼ cup

LEGUMES, PULSES, NUTS, AND SEEDS (CONT.)

GOS (CONT.)

Hazelnuts	10 nuts
Caraway seeds	2 tsp
Almond meal	¼ cup
Lentils, green or red, boiled	¼ cup
Chickpea pasta	1 cup
Red rice	1 cup

FRUCTANS

Chia seeds	2 Tbsp
Sunflower seeds	2 oz

CONDIMENTS, HERBS, SPICES, ETC.

GOS

Ketchup, sweetened with high fructose corn syrup	1 sachet
Fish sauce	1 Tbsp

FRUCTANS

Miso paste	2 Tbsp
Tahini	1 Tbsp

FRUCTOSE

Balsamic vinegar	1 Tbsp

CONFECTIONERY

FRUCTOSE

Honey	1 tsp
Agave syrup	1 tsp
Coconut sugar (also high in: fructans)	1 tsp

GOS

Dark chocolate, 85% or higher	5 squares

LACTOSE

Milk chocolate	4 squares

TOLERATED IN UNLIMITED AMOUNTS (TRACE OR NO FODMAPS)

GRAINS

Buckwheat groats
Arrowroot flour
Corn starch
Quinoa flour
Rice flour
Vermicelli noodles
Nutritional yeast flakes
Polenta
Brown rice
White rice

VEGETABLES

Arugula
Bean sprouts
Red bell pepper
Carrots
Collard greens
Cucumber
Endive, leaves
Ginger root
Kale
Romaine lettuce
Butter lettuce
Iceberg lettuce
Olives, black and green
Scallions, green tops
Parsnips
Potato
Radish
Seaweed, nori
Swiss chard
Tomato

FRUITS

Clementines
Dragonfruit
Grapes (red, black, white)
Guava, ripe
Mandarins
Navel oranges
Papaya
Prickly pear
Plantain
Rhubarb
Strawberries

DAIRY

Hard cheese, such as mozzarella, cheddar, and feta
Lactose-free milk
Lactose-free cottage cheese
Lactose-free sour cream
Lactose-free yogurt
Almond milk

LEGUMES, PULSES, NUTS, AND SEEDS

Macadamia nuts
Peanuts
Pecans
Pine nuts
Walnuts
Brazil nuts

WHY CANNED?
Once canned, beans and legumes lose some of their FODMAP content, so they often have lower levels of FODMAPs than dry varieties.

Elimination Phase Chart

TOLERATED IN UNLIMITED AMOUNTS (TRACE OR NO FODMAPS)

CONDIMENTS, HERBS, SPICES, ETC.

Butter
Mayo
Avocado oil
Canola oil
Coconut oil
Olive oil
Basil
Chili powder
Cilantro
Cinnamon
Cloves
Mint
Mustard
Paprika
Black pepper
Soy sauce
Apple cider vinegar

CONFECTIONERY

Stevia
Brown sugar
White sugar
Maple syrup
Vanilla essence
Sucralose

BEVERAGES

Beer
Cranberry juice
Espresso, black
Gin
Vodka
Red and white wine
Matcha tea
Green tea
Whiskey
Peppermint tea

10 Little Tricks That Can Help Promote Healthy Digestion

No matter how you modify the plan, be sure to practice these handy tips for minimizing stomach discomfort.

1 | Avoid chewing gum. Even if it doesn't contain sugar alcohols, it's bringing excess air into your body, which can cause bloating.

2 | Breathe! Improper breathing will lead to improper digestion.

3 | Calm down. Take deep breaths and relax before you eat.

4 | Eat slowly. Put your fork down between bites. Chew your food well.

5 | Sit down to eat. You're more likely to rush through your meal if you're not seated and settled comfortably. Pull up a chair and savor each bite!

6 | Exercise regularly. Physical activity helps the digestive system stay in check. Just make sure it's not too soon after eating.

7 | Drink water. But not too much before, with, or after meals to avoid bloating.

8 | Listen to hunger cues. Start eating when you feel hungry not "starved," and stop when you're satisfied not stuffed.

9 | Allow adequate time for digestion prior to bed. Try to give yourself 3 hours to digest a meal before going to sleep.

10 | Watch out for bubbles. Minimize or avoid carbonated beverages. (Mirkin says ½ Spindrift is an exception to the rule because it has very light carbonation and is low-FODMAP.)

Ready to start the meal plan? Turn the page for shopping lists and daily menus to get you through the next 3 weeks!

Master Meal Prep

Making healthy decisions is so much easier when they're right there in front of you! Mirkin suggests meal prepping as much as possible to limit time spent in the kitchen. Try making all breakfast and lunch recipes for the first half of the week on Sunday and prepping the remaining breakfasts and lunches on Wednesday.

Read all nutrition labels to make sure all packaged goods are free of sneaky high-FODMAP ingredients listed on page 14.

MEAT & PROTEIN

- ❏ 1 dozen eggs
- ❏ 1 32-oz carton liquid egg whites
- ❏ 3 oz chicken breast
- ❏ 4 oz ground beef extra-lean (97% lean)
- ❏ 4 oz ground chicken
- ❏ 1½ lbs 93% lean ground turkey
- ❏ 1 6-oz pkg. organic turkey bacon
- ❏ 12 oz (with bone) pork chop
- ❏ ½ lb scallops, fresh or frozen
- ❏ 9 oz shrimp
- ❏ 2 3-oz cans or pouches tuna fish
- ❏ 1 7-oz pkg. turkey deli meat
- ❏ 2 4-oz fillets wild salmon

PRODUCE

- ❏ 2 medium avocados
- ❏ 3 baby bell peppers
- ❏ 2 large red bell peppers
- ❏ 2 large green bell peppers
- ❏ 1 16-oz pkg. baby carrots
- ❏ 2 baby cucumbers
- ❏ 1 5-oz pkg. baby kale
- ❏ 2 large heads broccoli
- ❏ 1 cup cantaloupe
- ❏ 1 8-oz container cherry tomatoes
- ❏ 6 small tomatoes
- ❏ 13 medium tomatoes
- ❏ 1 small bunch fresh cilantro
- ❏ 1 small eggplant
- ❏ 1 small bunch fresh basil leaves
- ❏ 1 cup fresh pineapple
- ❏ 1 10-oz bag baby spinach
- ❏ 15 grapes
- ❏ 2 bunches scallions
- ❏ 2 kiwis
- ❏ 1 10-oz bag baby romaine lettuce
- ❏ 1 head butter lettuce
- ❏ 1 head large red romaine lettuce leaves
- ❏ 1 head iceberg lettuce
- ❏ 1 lime
- ❏ 1 16-oz bag mixed greens (including baby spinach, baby kale, mesclun, and arugula)
- ❏ 2 oranges
- ❏ 3 small white potatoes

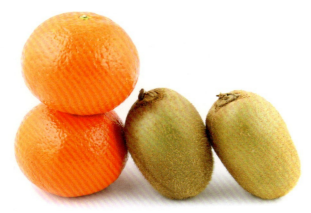

- ❏ 1 small container raspberries
- ❏ 1 medium spaghetti squash
- ❏ 1 16-oz container strawberries
- ❏ 1 tangerine
- ❏ 1 yellow squash
- ❏ 1 14-oz pkg. frozen spinach

DAIRY

- ❏ 1 6-oz pkg. Cheddar cheese slices
- ❏ 1 6-oz pkg. Colby Jack cheese slices
- ❏ 1 6-oz container feta cheese
- ❏ 2 16-oz containers lactose-free cottage cheese
- ❏ 1 pint 1% lactose-free milk
- ❏ 1 6-oz container lactose-free yogurt
- ❏ 1 8-oz container grated Parmesan cheese
- ❏ 1 6-oz container part-skim ricotta cheese
- ❏ 1 8-oz pkg. shredded Cheddar cheese
- ❏ 1 8-oz container sour cream
- ❏ 1 12-oz pkg. string cheese

PANTRY

- ❏ 1 5-oz bag almonds (or smallest available)
- ❏ 1 small bottle avocado oil
- ❏ 1 avocado oil spray
- ❏ 1 bottle balsamic vinegar
- ❏ 1 pkg. brown rice tortilla
- ❏ 1 pkg. whole-grain corn tortilla sliders
- ❏ 1 jar canola mayonnaise
- ❏ 1 8-oz bag chia seeds
- ❏ 1 box chickpea pasta

- ❏ 1 bottle ground cinnamon
- ❏ 1 bar dark chocolate (at least 85% cocoa)
- ❏ 1 medium bag dark chocolate almonds
- ❏ 1 8-oz jar Dijon mustard
- ❏ 1 bottle dried basil
- ❏ 1 bottle dried oregano
- ❏ 1 bottle extra virgin olive oil
- ❏ 1 8-oz pkg. firm tofu
- ❏ 1 bottle garlic-infused oil (or use recipe on p. 14)
- ❏ 1 loaf gluten-free whole-grain bread
- ❏ 1 container Kosher salt
- ❏ 1 can lentils
- ❏ 1 bottle low-FODMAP salad dressing (or use recipe on p.104)
- ❏ 1 container nutritional yeast
- ❏ 1 pkg. old-fashioned rolled oats
- ❏ 1 jar natural peanut butter
- ❏ 1 container ground black pepper
- ❏ 1 6-oz bag pumpkin seeds
- ❏ 1 bottle pure vanilla extract
- ❏ 1 bottle reduced-sodium soy sauce
- ❏ 1 container sea salt
- ❏ 1 bottle shallot-infused oil (or use recipe on p.14)
- ❏ 1 jar sunflower seed butter
- ❏ 1 6-oz bag sunflower seeds
- ❏ 1 bottle turmeric
- ❏ 1 6-oz bag walnuts
- ❏ 1 28-oz can whole peeled tomatoes

DAY 1

BREAKFAST

Cheesy Omelet

Heat skillet on medium and coat with a light layer of avocado oil spray. In a medium bowl, mix 1 egg, ½ cup egg whites, 1 Tbsp lactose-free milk, and a dash of salt and pepper. Add to skillet and allow to set, then flip and add 2 cups spinach, ¼ cup chopped scallion tips, and 1 Tbsp shredded Cheddar cheese. Remove from burner after a few minutes and top with Low-FODMAP Salsa (p. 103) or 1 small chopped tomato, 2 scallion tips, chopped cilantro, and a squeeze of lime juice.

SNACK

String Cheese and Carrots

1 stick string cheese

⅓ cup baby carrots

LUNCH

Open-Faced Turkey and Cheese

In a toaster oven, toast 1 slice gluten-free whole-grain bread such as Udi's (check that it doesn't include added honey, inulin, or concentrated fruit juice). Once bread is lightly browned, add 2 leaves lettuce, 3 oz turkey, and 1 slice Cheddar cheese and continue toasting until cheese melts. Top with tomato slices. Enjoy with 1 orange.

SNACK

Tuna Salad

In a small bowl, mix one 3-oz pouch tuna (Mirkin likes Safe Catch, which is a low-mercury option) with 1 Tbsp canola mayo and 1 chopped scallion tip. Scoop into large romaine lettuce leaves.

DINNER

Lentil and Beef Burgers in Lettuce Wraps (p. 61)

Serve with ¾ cup steamed broccoli topped with 1 Tbsp Parmesan cheese.

SNACK

Dark Chocolate Almonds

10 dark chocolate–covered almonds, at least 85% cocoa

NUTRITION (per day): 1,543 cal, 129 g pro, 109 g carb, 25 g fiber, 44 g sugars (2 g added sugars), 70 g fat (24 sat fat), 412 mg chol, 1,360 mg sodium

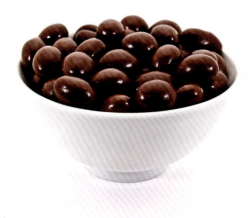

DAY 2

BREAKFAST

High-Protein Oatmeal (p.62)

SNACK

Turkey Cheese Wraps

Wrap 1 slice turkey around 1 stick string cheese, then wrap in large lettuce leaf. Top with Dijon mustard and eat with 6 cherry tomatoes.

LUNCH

Leftover Lentil and Beef Burgers in Lettuce Wraps. Serve over 4 cups mix of baby spinach, baby kale, mesclun, and arugula tossed with 1 sliced medium beefsteak tomato, 1 sliced baby cucumber, 2 Tbsp sliced avocado, and 2 Tbsp low-FODMAP dressing.

SNACK

Cottage Cheese and Berries

Top ½ cup lactose-free cottage cheese with ½ cup strawberries and dash of cinnamon.

DINNER

Ground Turkey Calzone (p. 65)

SNACK

Chocolate and Peanut Butter

Top 1 square extra-dark chocolate with 2 tsp peanut butter.

NUTRITION (per day): 1,700 cal, 139 g pro, 156 g carb, 37 g fiber, 52 g sugars (2 g added sugars), 66 g fat (20 g sat fat), 216 mg chol, 2,126 mg sodium

DAY 3

BREAKFAST

Yogurt and Berries

Top 6 oz lactose-free yogurt with 2 Tbsp chia seeds, 1 Tbsp chopped walnuts, and 1 cup sliced strawberries.

SNACK

Simple Chicken Taco

Heat 1 corn tortilla slider in the microwave or in a small skillet until warm. Top with 1 oz chicken breast, Low-FODMAP Salsa, 2 or 3 torn romaine lettuce leaves, and 1 Tbsp sour cream (low-FODMAP taco sauce optional).

LUNCH

Leftover Ground Turkey Calzone

SNACK

Fruit and Cheese

1 tangerine and 1 stick string cheese.

DINNER

Pork Chops (p. 66)

SNACK

Carrots and Sunflower Seed Butter

⅓ cup baby carrots dipped in 1 Tbsp sunflower seed butter.

NUTRITION (per day): 1,538 cal, 117 g pro, 104 g carb, 28 g fiber, 62 g sugars (1 g added sugars), 78 g fat (24 g sat fat), 216 mg chol, 1070 mg sodium

DAY 4

BREAKFAST

Tofu Scramble with Diced Tomato and Avocado (p. 69)

SNACK

Cottage Cheese and Fruit

½ cup lactose-free cottage cheese with 1 cup fresh pineapple.

LUNCH

Leftover Pork Chops

SNACK

Melty Chicken Wrap

Heat a medium skillet over medium-high and lightly coat with avocado oil spray. Cook ½ brown rice tortilla in skillet until browned on both sides. Remove from pan and top with 2 Tbsp avocado, 2 oz cooked chicken breast, 3 leaves lettuce, 2 Tbsp chopped scallion tips, and 1 small tomato, chopped.

Tip: If you buy packaged turkey or chicken, make sure it doesn't contain honey, which is high-FODMAP, or any nitrates or celery powder, which are thought to increase cancer risk.

DINNER

Scallop Salad (p. 71)

SNACK

Dark Chocolate Almonds

10 dark chocolate–covered almonds, at least 85% cocoa.

NUTRITION (per day): 1,749 cal, 89 g pro, 120 g carb, 29 g fiber, 53 g sugars (0 g added sugars), 109 g fat (16 g sat fat), 200 mg chol, 1,150 mg sodium

DAY 5

BREAKFAST

Egg White Omelet

Heat ½ tsp shallot-infused oil on medium-high. Add 1 cup egg whites with 2 cups spinach and ¼ cup shredded Cheddar. Top with 1 cup Low-FODMAP Salsa. Serve with ½ cup lactose-free cottage cheese.

SNACK

Leftover Scallops

Enjoy 4 leftover scallops over 2 cups mixed greens with 1 Tbsp low-FODMAP dressing.

LUNCH

Open-Faced Tuna Salad Sandwich

Mix 3 oz tuna fish with 1 Tbsp canola mayonnaise and ¼ cup chopped scallion. Spread on 1 slice toasted gluten-free whole-grain bread. Top with 2 slices medium tomato and 1 slice melted Cheddar. Enjoy with 2 kiwis.

SNACK

Cottage Cheese with Peanut Butter and Berries

Mix 1 Tbsp peanut butter with ¼ cup lactose-free cottage cheese and ½ cup heated strawberries.

DINNER

Protein Pasta (p. 72)

SNACK

Ricotta Cheese with Berries

Mix 2 Tbsp part-skim ricotta cheese with 10 raspberries.

NUTRITION (per day): 1,723 cal, 144 g pro, 133 g carb, 30 g fiber, 28 g sugars (2 g added sugars), 70 g fat (16 g sat fat), 165 mg chol, 2,400 mg sodium

DAY 6

BREAKFAST

2 Egg Muffins (p. 75)
Enjoy with ½ cup lactose-free cottage cheese and 1 cup cantaloupe.

SNACK

Leftover Protein Pasta (½ serving)

LUNCH

Feta and Shrimp Salad
Top 4 cups mixed greens with 4 oz cooked shrimp, 2 Tbsp avocado, 1 small tomato (sliced), ⅓ cup scallion tips, 2 Tbsp feta cheese, and 2 Tbsp low-FODMAP dressing.

SNACK

Fruit and Pumpkin Seeds
1 orange with ¼ cup pumpkin seeds.

DINNER

Salmon Parmesan with Broccoli and Potato (p. 76)

SNACK

Fruit and Nuts
15 grapes and 10 walnut halves

NUTRITION (per day): 1,752 cal, 128 g pro, 152 g carb, 26 g fiber, 63 g sugars (0 g added sugars), 77 g fat (26 g sat fat), 638 mg chol, 2,040 mg sodium

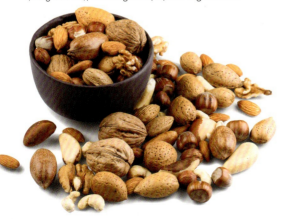

DAY 7

BREAKFAST

Avocado Egg Scramble
Mix 1 cup egg whites and 1 whole egg with a dash of sea salt and 1 Tbsp milk. Add to a skillet lightly coated with ½ tsp shallot-infused oil over medium heat. Mix with ½ cup cooked spinach and top with 2 Tbsp avocado and Low-FODMAP Salsa.

SNACK

Leftover Protein Pasta (½ serving)

LUNCH

Sarah's Turkey Burger (p. 79)

SNACK

Egg Muffin and Peppers
1 egg muffin with 3 baby bell peppers.

DINNER

Shrimp Squash Pasta
Cut medium-size spaghetti squash in half. Steam open side face down in a pot filled halfway with boiling water. Scoop out seeds. Mix 3 cups cooked spaghetti squash with 5 oz cooked shrimp, 2 tsp garlic-infused oil (p. 14 or use Fody Foods Garlic Infused Extra Virgin Olive Oil), a dash of sea salt, and 2 Tbsp Parmesan cheese. Serve with 2 cups baby kale sautéed in 1 tsp garlic-infused oil.

SNACK

Chocolate Peanut Butter Crunch
Dip 1 dark chocolate square in ½ Tbsp peanut butter mixed with 1 tsp chia seeds.

NUTRITION (per day): 1,723 cal, 124 g pro, 93 g carb, 31 g fiber, 36 g sugars (0 g added sugars), 102 g fat (20 g sat fat), 730 mg chol, 2,300 mg sodium

Read all nutrition labels to make sure all packaged goods are free of sneaky high-FODMAP ingredients listed on page 14. Check for leftover ingredients from Week 1 before purchasing new ingredients from the shopping list.

MEAT & PROTEIN

- ❏ 1 3-oz can or pouch tuna fish
- ❏ 2 lbs chicken breast
- ❏ 2 dozen eggs
- ❏ 1 16-oz container liquid egg whites
- ❏ 1 lb ground turkey (93% lean)
- ❏ 1 6-oz pkg. organic turkey bacon
- ❏ 2 oz shrimp
- ❏ 1 lb sirloin steak
- ❏ 3 oz smoked salmon
- ❏ 1⅓ lbs fresh wild salmon

PRODUCE

- ❏ 1 5-oz bag power greens (includes baby kale, baby spinach, chard, and mizuna)
- ❏ 3 5-oz bags arugula
- ❏ 2 large avocados
- ❏ 3 red bell peppers
- ❏ 4 baby bell peppers
- ❏ 1 16-oz bag or 1 ½ cups baby carrots
- ❏ 2 large carrots
- ❏ 1 head romaine lettuce leaves
- ❏ 1 5-oz bag baby romaine
- ❏ ½ cantaloupe
- ❏ 1 16-oz container cherry tomatoes
- ❏ 10 medium tomatoes
- ❏ 2 medium cucumbers
- ❏ 1 small bunch fresh dill
- ❏ 1 14-oz pkg. frozen spinach
- ❏ 1 10-oz bag baby spinach
- ❏ 1 small bag grapes

- ❏ 15 green beans
- ❏ 3 bunches scallions
- ❏ 2 kiwis
- ❏ 1 lemon
- ❏ 2 medium zucchinis
- ❏ 1 5-oz bag mixed greens
- ❏ 1 navel orange
- ❏ 5 large olives
- ❏ 1 small bunch oregano leaves
- ❏ 1 small ripe papaya
- ❏ 1 small bunch parsley
- ❏ 1 9-oz potato
- ❏ 1 radish
- ❏ 1 6-oz container raspberries
- ❏ 2 12-oz containers strawberries (minimum if 2 strawberries are leftover from previous week)

DAIRY

- ❏ 1 stick butter
- ❏ 1 8-oz pkg. Cheddar cheese
- ❏ 1 small container feta cheese
- ❏ 1 16-oz container lactose-free cottage cheese
- ❏ 1 pint 1% lactose-free milk
- ❏ 1 8-oz container grated Parmesan cheese
- ❏ 1 8-oz container whipped cream cheese

PANTRY

- ❏ 1 bottle bay leaves
- ❏ 1 small can black beans
- ❏ 1 box brown rice crackers
- ❏ 1 pkg. medium whole-grain corn tortillas
- ❏ 1 small container brown sugar
- ❏ 1 8-oz block extra-firm tofu
- ❏ 1 bag frozen hash brown potatoes, plain
- ❏ 1 bottle low-FODMAP Caesar dressing
- ❏ 1 bottle low-FODMAP ketchup
- ❏ 1 container unsweetened pea protein powder (no added gums or sweeteners)
- ❏ 1 small container pecans
- ❏ 1 bottle rice vinegar
- ❏ 1 small can tomato paste
- ❏ 1 3-oz pkg. slivered almonds

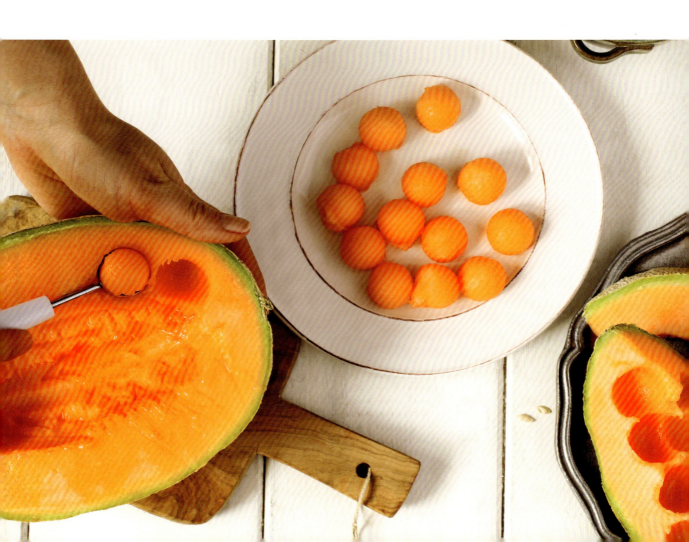

DAY 8

BREAKFAST

Breakfast Quesadillas

Warm 2 whole-grain corn tortilla sliders in a pan lightly coated with butter. Flip after 30 seconds and add ½ slice cheese to each. Cook until cheese is slightly melted, then remove from heat. Heat 2 Tbsp rinsed, canned black beans. Add beans, chopped tomatoes, and handful of arugula to tortillas. Fold and eat!

SNACK

2 Egg Muffins (p. 75)

LUNCH

Caesar Chicken Wraps (p. 80)

SNACK

Fruit and Cheese

2 kiwis with 1 oz Colby or Cheddar cheese.

DINNER

Salmon and Green Beans

In a medium skillet over medium, heat 1 tsp garlic-infused oil. Add 6 oz wild salmon coated with dash of salt and pepper, and sautée for 4 to 5 minutes per side. In a nonstick pan or microwave, cook 15 green beans for 6 to 8 minutes, or until desired tenderness.

SNACK

Chocolate Raspberry Ricotta

In a small saucepan over medium, heat 7 raspberries until a compote starts to form. Pour over 2 Tbsp ricotta cheese. Top with 1 Tbsp dark chocolate nibs.

NUTRITION (per day): 1,635 cal, 120 g pro, 94 g carb, 28 g fiber, 20 g sugars (1 g added sugars), 89 g fat (26 g sat fat), 558 mg chol, 1,110 mg sodium

DAY 9

BREAKFAST

Hard-Boiled Eggs with Fruit

3 hard-boiled eggs with 1 navel orange.

SNACK

Leftover Caesar Chicken Wrap (½ serving)

LUNCH

Turkey Spinach Salad

Toss 3 cups spinach and mixed greens with 2 Tbsp avocado, ⅓ cup shredded carrots, 1 chopped tomato, ½ cup cucumber slices, and 1 Tbsp feta cheese. Top with 1 leftover turkey burger cut into bite-size pieces and 2 Tbsp low-FODMAP dressing.

Tip: When reheating the turkey burger, add water to maintain moisture.

SNACK

Leftover Egg Muffin and Peppers

1 egg muffin cup and 4 baby bell peppers.

DINNER

Salmon Burgers (p. 83)

SNACK

Chocolate

1 oz dark chocolate (at least 85% cocoa)

NUTRITION (per day): 1,682 cal, 121 g pro, 78 g carb, 19 g fiber, 41 g sugars (0 g added sugars), 100 g fat (31 g sat fat), 1,100 mg chol, 1,320 mg sodium

DAY 10

BREAKFAST

Toast and Smoked Salmon
Top 1 slice gluten-free whole-grain toast with 2 Tbsp whipped cream cheese, 3 oz nitrate-free smoked salmon, and 1 cup arugula.

SNACK

Cottage Cheese and Fruit
1½ cups papaya with ½ cup lactose-free cottage cheese.

LUNCH

Chicken Strawberry Salad
Toss 3 cups spinach with 6 oz chicken breast, ½ cup strawberries, 2 Tbsp slivered almonds, 1 Tbsp rice vinegar, and 1 Tbsp avocado or olive oil.

SNACK

Leftover Caesar Chicken Wraps (½ serving)

DINNER

Leftover Salmon Burgers

SNACK

Chocolate Peanut Butter Crunch
Dip 1 dark chocolate square in 1 Tbsp peanut butter mixed with 1 Tbsp chia seeds.

NUTRITION (per day): 1,638 cal, 136 g pro, 89 g carb, 24 g fiber, 56 g sugars (0 g added sugars), 185 g fat (20 g sat fat), 230 mg chol, 2,100 mg sodium

DAY 11

BREAKFAST

Bacon Breakfast Wrap
Heat 1 brown rice wrap in a skillet over medium. Top with 2 oz turkey bacon, 1 over-easy egg, 1 slice Colby cheese, ¼ cup arugula, ¼ cup baby romaine, and ½ cup diced tomatoes.

SNACK

Tuna Salad
Mix 3 oz canned tuna fish with 1 Tbsp olive or canola oil-based mayonnaise and 1 scallion tip. Serve in ½ small cantaloupe, seeds scooped out (1 cup).

LUNCH

Greek Salad
Toss 4 cups romaine lettuce with 5 olives, 4 oz chicken breast, 2 Tbsp avocado, ¼ cup scallion tips, 6 sliced cherry tomatoes, 2 Tbsp feta cheese, 2 tsp olive oil, and 2 tsp balsamic vinegar.

SNACK

Crackers and Cheese
5 brown rice crackers with 1 slice hard cheese and ½ cup cherry tomatoes.

DINNER

Beef Stew (p. 85)

SNACK

Cottage Cheese and Fruit
Mix ¼ cup lactose-free cottage cheese with 1 tsp peanut butter, 10 raspberries, and 1 tsp chia seeds.

NUTRITION (per day): 1,798 cal, 139 g pro, 123 g carb, 28 g fiber, 38 g sugars (0 g added sugars), 85 g fat (33 g sat fat), 570 mg chol, 1,975 mg sodium

DAY 12

BREAKFAST

Smoothie Bowl

Lightly blend 1 cup lactose-free 1% milk with 1½ cups strawberries, 1 Tbsp chia seeds, and 1 scoop pea protein powder. Serve in a bowl.

SNACK

Tomato Cheese Melt

Cut 1 beefsteak tomato in half. Top each half with ½ oz Cheddar and heat for about 20 seconds in microwave or until cheese melts.

LUNCH

Leftover Beef Stew (1 serving)

SNACK

Hard-Boiled Eggs and Veggies

2 hard-boiled eggs with ½ cup sliced cucumber.

DINNER

Marinated Tofu Salad (p. 87)

SNACK

Dark Chocolate

1 square dark chocolate with 1 cup lactose-free 1% milk.

NUTRITION (per day): 1,731 cal, 173 g pro, 106 g carb, 24 g fiber, 53 g sugars (4 g added sugars), 72 g fat (21 g sat fat), 520 mg chol, 1,350 mg sodium

DAY 13

BREAKFAST

Eggs and Potatoes

2 eggs over easy with ½ cup hash brown potatoes prepared with 1 tsp oil and a dash of salt and pepper, with 1 Tbsp low-FODMAP ketchup and 1½ cups mixed fruit (strawberries, grapes, blueberries, cantaloupe, papaya).

SNACK

Cheesy Quesadilla

1 corn tortilla slider or ½ regular-size corn tortilla heated on burner and filled with 1 Tbsp shredded Cheddar, 1 Tbsp black beans, Low-FODMAP Salsa, and arugula (taco sauce optional).

LUNCH

Chicken Spinach Salad

Toss 4 cups spinach with 4 oz chicken breast, 6 walnut halves, 4 sliced strawberries, 2 Tbsp feta cheese, and 2 Tbsp low-FODMAP dressing.

SNACK

Pumpkin Seeds

¼ cup pumpkin seeds.

DINNER

Pecan-Crusted Salmon Salad (p. 88)

SNACK

Cheese and Fruit

1 oz cheese with 1 cup grapes.

NUTRITION (per day): 1,590 cal, 114 g pro, 104 g carb, 19 g fiber, 42 g sugars (2 g added sugars), 85 g fat (21 g sat fat), 750 mg chol, 1,450 mg sodium

DAY 14

BREAKFAST

Zucchini, Bell Pepper, and Feta Frittata
(1½ servings) (p. 91)
Top with 2 Tbsp sour cream and Low-FODMAP Salsa.

SNACK

Shrimp Taco
In a small skillet, heat 1 whole-grain corn tortilla. Fill with 2 cooked medium shrimp, 2 Tbsp avocado, and Low-FODMAP Salsa.

LUNCH

Leftover Marinated Tofu Salad

SNACK

Cottage Cheese and Fruit
Top ½ cup lactose-free cottage cheese with ½ cup strawberries, warmed either in the microwave or a skillet. Add a dash of cinnamon and 1 tsp pecan pieces.

DINNER

Italian Turkey Meatloaf with Arugula Salad
(p. 92)

SNACK

Fruit and Nuts
15 walnut halves and 15 grapes.

NUTRITION (per day): 1,542 cal, 117 g pro, 90 g carb, 26 g fiber, 35 g sugars (2 g added sugars), 85 g fat (16 g sat fat), 420 mg chol, 1,400 mg sodium

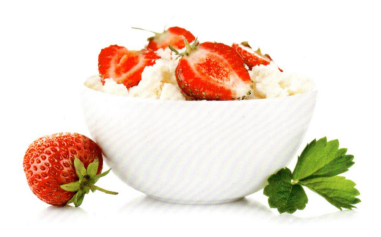

Read all nutrition labels to make sure all packaged goods are free of sneaky high-FODMAP ingredients listed on page 14. Check for leftover ingredients from Week 2 before purchasing new ingredients from the shopping list.

MEAT & PROTEIN

- ❑ 14 oz chicken breast, raw
- ❑ 6 oz cooked chicken breast
- ❑ ½ dozen eggs
- ❑ 1 16-oz container liquid egg whites
- ❑ 3 oz 93% lean ground sirloin
- ❑ 1 lb ground turkey
- ❑ 6 oz salmon
- ❑ 5 oz smoked salmon
- ❑ 12 oz shrimp
- ❑ 6 oz sole
- ❑ 1 8-oz pkg. tempeh
- ❑ 6 oz turkey breast meat

PRODUCE

- ❑ 1 5-oz bag arugula
- ❑ 1 small avocado
- ❑ 1 10-oz bag baby spinach
- ❑ 1 bunch or 3 small pkgs. fresh basil
- ❑ 3 red bell peppers
- ❑ 1 16-oz container blueberries
- ❑ 2 carrots
- ❑ 1 16-oz container cherry tomatoes
- ❑ 3 medium tomatoes
- ❑ 2 large tomatoes
- ❑ ¼ cup corn (frozen, canned, or fresh)

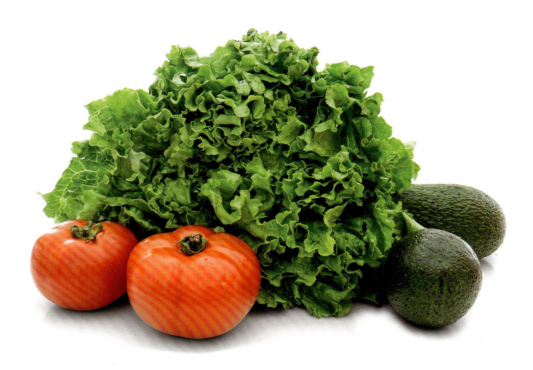

- ❏ 2 small cucumbers
- ❏ 1 small eggplant
- ❏ 1 small piece ginger
- ❏ 15 green beans
- ❏ 3 bunches scallions
- ❏ 3 heads romaine lettuce
- ❏ 1 head iceberg lettuce
- ❏ 2 lemons
- ❏ 1 lime
- ❏ 2 kiwis
- ❏ 20 large olives
- ❏ 1 10-oz bag mixed greens (baby spinach and baby kale mix)
- ❏ 4 oranges
- ❏ ½ cup fresh oyster mushrooms
- ❏ 1 small papaya
- ❏ ¾ cup pineapple
- ❏ 1 3-oz potato
- ❏ 1 small container raspberries
- ❏ 1 spaghetti squash
- ❏ 1 12-oz container strawberries
- ❏ 1 10-oz pkg. frozen strawberries
- ❏ 1 zucchini

DAIRY

- ❏ 1 stick butter
- ❏ 1 16-oz container lactose-free cottage cheese
- ❏ 1 pint 1% lactose-free milk
- ❏ 1 6-oz container lactose-free yogurt
- ❏ 1 8-oz bag shredded Mexican-style cheese
- ❏ 1 small container mozzarella cheese
- ❏ 1 can whipped cream

PANTRY

- ❏ 1 pkg. brown rice cakes
- ❏ 1 small can black beans
- ❏ 1 small bottle capers
- ❏ 1 bottle dried marjoram
- ❏ 1 bottle dried rosemary
- ❏ 1 bottle dried sage
- ❏ 1 bottle dried thyme
- ❏ 1 8-oz block firm tofu
- ❏ 1 small pkg. frozen strawberries
- ❏ 1 small can chickpeas
- ❏ 1 small bottle horseradish
- ❏ 1 bottle red pepper flakes
- ❏ 1 bottle low-FODMAP taco sauce (FODY brand)
- ❏ 1 bottle low-FODMAP taco seasoning (FODY brand)
- ❏ 1 small container pine nuts
- ❏ 1 small pkg. tapioca starch
- ❏ 1 loaf gluten-free whole-grain bread

DAY 15

BREAKFAST

Leftover Zucchini, Bell Pepper, and Feta Frittata (1½ servings)

Top with Low-FODMAP Salsa and 2 Tbsp sour cream.

SNACK

Fruit and Nuts

15 almonds with 2 kiwis.

LUNCH

Leftover Italian Turkey Meatloaf

SNACK

Rice Cake and Sunflower Seed Butter

Top 1 brown rice cake with 1 Tbsp sunflower seed butter.

DINNER

Shrimp Tacos with Sautéed Spinach (p. 95)

SNACK

Dark Chocolate and Fruit

1 cup frozen strawberries with 1 square dark chocolate.

NUTRITION (per day): 1,566 cal, 101 g pro, 101 g carb, 28 g fiber, 35 g sugars (0 g added sugars), 89 g fat (26 g sat fat), 780 mg chol, 1,500 mg sodium

DAY 16

BREAKFAST

High-Protein Oatmeal (p. 62)

Swap 1 Tbsp chia seeds with 1 Tbsp peanut butter and swap ½ cup strawberries for ¼ heaping cup blueberries.

SNACK

Leftover Italian Turkey Meatloaf (½ serving)

Wrap in lettuce leaves with 2 Tbsp avocado.

LUNCH

Shrimp Salad

Toss 5 oz leftover shrimp with 4 cups mixed greens, 5 sliced olives, 10 sliced cherry tomatoes, ¼ cup scallion tips, 1 Tbsp feta, and 2 Tbsp low-FODMAP dressing.

SNACK

Cottage Cheese and Fruit

¾ cup pineapple with ⅓ cup lactose-free cottage cheese.

DINNER

Chicken Margherita (p. 96)

SNACK

Chocolate Berries and Cream

Top ¼ cup blueberries and ¾ cup strawberries with 1 tsp chocolate nibs and 2 Tbsp whipped cream.

NUTRITION (per day): 1,582 cal, 131 g pro, 116 g carb, 24 g fiber, 53 g sugars (0 g added sugars), 72 g fat (21 g sat fat), 420 mg chol, 1,742 mg sodium

DAY 17

BREAKFAST

Tofu Scramble with Diced Tomato and Avocado (p. 69)
Substitute avocado with 5 olives.

SNACK

Peanut Butter and Berry Toast
Top 1 slice low-FODMAP bread with 1 Tbsp peanut butter and 2 sliced strawberries (heat the berries to make them sweeter).

LUNCH

Leftover Chicken Margherita
Serve over 4 cups mixed greens.

SNACK

Meatloaf Wrap
Wrap ½ portion leftover turkey meatloaf in large lettuce leaves with 2 Tbsp avocado.

DINNER

Baked Sole with Veggies and Potato
Heat oven to 375°F. Place 6 oz sole in a baking dish and top with a squeeze of lemon, 1 tsp capers, 2 chopped scallion tips, and 1 Tbsp garlic-infused oil. Cook for 8 to 10 minutes, or until fish flakes easily. Serve over bed of arugula with 1 3-oz potato.

SNACK

Berry Crepe
In a small skillet lightly coated with butter over medium, cook 2 egg whites so they form a thin shell. Fill the shell with 2 Tbsp lactose-free cottage cheese, and ¼ cup heated blueberries. Top with cinnamon.

NUTRITION (per day): 1,608 cal, 125 g pro, 92 g carb, 26 g fiber, 22 g sugars (0 g added sugars), 87 g fat (8 g sat fat), 180 mg chol, 1,200 mg sodium

DAY 18

BREAKFAST

Smoked Salmon Breakfast Wrap
In a small skillet lightly coated with butter, heat 1 brown rice wrap on medium until lightly browned, about 1 minute per side. Fill with 1 Tbsp cream cheese, 3 oz smoked salmon, dash of scallion tips, and handful of arugula.

SNACK

Yogurt Bowl
Top 6 oz lactose-free yogurt with 1 Tbsp chia seeds and 10 blueberries.

LUNCH

Chopped Chicken Salad
Chop 6 oz cooked chicken breast, 1 small cucumber, ½ red bell pepper, 4 cups romaine lettuce, 1 medium tomato, 5 large olives, and ¼ cup chickpeas. Toss together with 2 Tbsp low-FODMAP dressing.

SNACK

Fruit and Nuts
15 almonds with 1 orange.

DINNER

Tempeh in Lettuce Leaves (p. 99)

SNACK

Dark Chocolate
2 dark chocolate squares.

NUTRITION (per day): 1,547 cal, 106 g pro, 137 g carb, 29 g fiber, 50 g sugars (6 g added sugars), 70 g fat (19 g sat fat), 160 mg chol, 1,950 mg sodium

DAY 19

BREAKFAST

Smoothie Bowl

Blend 1 cup lactose-free milk, ¼ cup blueberries, ½ cup strawberries, 2 Tbsp chia seeds, ice, and 1 scoop pea protein powder until smooth. Serve in bowl and eat with spoon.

SNACK

Turkey and Cucumber

Wrap 2 oz turkey around ½ cucumber with Dijon mustard. Eat with 1 orange.

LUNCH

Leftover Tempeh in Lettuce Leaves

Enjoy with 1 cup papaya.

SNACK

Cottage Cheese–Stuffed Pepper

Stuff ½ red bell pepper with ¼ cup lactose-free cottage cheese and dash of scallion tips.

DINNER

Sheet Pan Chicken Pesto Primavera

Heat oven to 400°F. Place 6 oz chicken breast, ½ sliced zucchini, and ½ sliced eggplant (about 1 cup) on a large sheet pan and toss with 1 tsp olive oil and ½ Tbsp pesto (p. 103). Bake for 10 minutes. Remove from oven and drain excess liquid. Add ½ cup oyster mushrooms and another Tbsp pesto. Toss to combine, then bake another 10 minutes until chicken is fully cooked.

SNACK

Sunflower Seeds

¼ cup sunflower seeds.

NUTRITION (per day): 1,508 cal, 127 g pro, 121 g carb, 30 g fiber, 48 g sugars (0 g added sugars), 66 g fat (10 g sat fat), 160 mg chol, 110 mg sodium

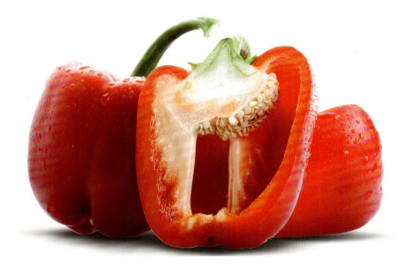

DAY 20

BREAKFAST

Mediterranean Omelet

In a medium skillet lightly coated with avocado oil, sautée 2 cups baby spinach, 5 sliced olives, and ¼ cup chopped tomatoes over medium-high until desired tenderness and set aside. In a separate pan, heat 1 tsp avocado oil over medium. Mix together 1 whole egg, ½ cup egg whites, 1 Tbsp lactose-free milk, and a dash of salt and pepper. Add egg mixture to pan. Once it sets, top with veggies and fold. Sprinkle with 2 Tbsp feta and enjoy!

SNACK

Loaded Rice Cakes

Top 1 rice cake with ¼ cup lactose-free cottage cheese, 6 raspberries, and cinnamon.

LUNCH

Taco Salad (p. 100)

SNACK

Simple Shrimp Cocktail

Mix 1 Tbsp low-FODMAP ketchup (such as Fody brand) with ¼ tsp horseradish to make your own low-FODMAP cocktail sauce. Enjoy with 6 cooked shrimp.

DINNER

Sautéed Beef and Spaghetti Squash

In a medium skillet lightly coated with avocado oil, cook 3 oz ground sirloin on medium-high, breaking meat apart with spatula, for approximately 6 to 8 minutes, until there is almost no pink left. Then add ½ cup low-FODMAP tomato sauce to the beef and simmer for about 4 minutes. At the same time, cut the spaghetti squash in half and steam open side down in a pot filled halfway with boiling water, or simply place in the microwave for 8 to 10 minutes. Remove the seeds and add the beef-tomato sauce mixture and top with 2 Tbsp Parmesan cheese.

SNACK

Sunflower Seed Butter Toast

Toast 1 slice gluten-free whole-grain bread and top with 1 Tbsp sunflower seed butter.

NUTRITION (per day): 1,558 cal, 124 g pro, 116 g carb, 26 g fiber, 33 g sugars (4 g added sugars), 72 g fat (21 g sat fat), 740 mg chol, 2,300 mg sodium

Store-Bought Low-FODMAP Foods

It can be difficult to determine whether a product is truly low-FODMAP. Here are some of Mirkin's favorite low-FODMAP go-tos available at most grocery stores or online:

Bread: Udi's Multigrain Sandwich Bread

Tortillas: Food For Life Brown Rice Tortillas

Salad Dressing: Fody Low-FODMAP Salad Dressings

Ketchup: Fody Low-FODMAP Ketchup

DAY 21

BREAKFAST

Smoked Salmon Roll

Make a wrap by mixing 1 egg and 1 egg white and cooking in a medium skillet lightly coated with butter over medium-high heat. Add 1 Tbsp cream cheese, scallion tips, 2 oz smoked salmon, and arugula. Wrap it up!

SNACK

Spaghetti Squash

Toss 2 cups leftover spaghetti squash with 1 tsp garlic-infused oil, a dash of salt, 6 cherry tomatoes (halved), and ¼ cup Parmesan cheese.

LUNCH

Brown Rice Turkey Wrap

In a medium skillet heated on medium-high, roll a stick of butter over the pan to lightly coat. Add a brown rice tortilla and cook about 30 to 60 seconds per side, or until lightly browned. Remove and plate. Add 2 Tbsp avocado, a dash of scallion tips, ½ cup sliced tomato, 3 oz turkey breast, and 1 Tbsp canola mayonnaise.

Tip: Wet the turkey with a little water and heat it in the pan once you remove the tortilla. This will keep it moist and hot.

SNACK

Leftover Taco Salad (½ serving)

DINNER

Baked Salmon with Green Beans and Carrots

Heat oven to 375°F. Coat a baking sheet with foil and add 6 oz salmon. In a small bowl, mix together 1 tsp garlic-infused oil, 2 Tbsp scallion tips, a dash of sea salt and black pepper, a squeeze of lemon, and ½ Tbsp fresh dill. Pour mixture over salmon and seal the foil. Bake approximately 15 minutes, or until salmon flakes easily with a fork. While the salmon is cooking, slice 1 carrot lengthwise. Steam the sliced carrot and 15 green beans in a steam basket or in the microwave approximately 6 to 8 minutes, depending on desired tenderness.

SNACK

Cheese and Fruit

1 stick string cheese with 2 oranges.

NUTRITION (per day): 1,544 cal, 117 g pro, 107 g carb, 27 g fiber, 35 g sugars (0 g added sugars), 78 g fat (20 g sat fat), 400 mg chol, 1,775 mg sodium

CHAPTER 5

The Reintroduction Phase

Now that you're symptom-free, you can start reintroducing FODMAPs into your diet. It may be tempting to skip this step and continue eating like you did during the elimination phase, especially if this is the first time you've enjoyed symptom-free days in a while. But it is critical to reintroduce FOD-MAPs into your diet so you can discover which ones you tolerate and build out a diverse and nutrient-rich diet from that point.

How to Reintroduce

Over the course of about 9 weeks, you will reintroduce a different FODMAP one at a time, one day at a time. Spend the day after each reintroduction eating only low-FODMAP. How your body responds on this day will determine what you do next:

- If you experience symptoms this day, continue eating low-FODMAP for a total of 3 days (or until symptoms disappear), then move on to reintroducing the next FODMAP.

- If you do not experience symptoms on this day, have a slightly larger serving of the FODMAP the fol-

lowing day. If you continue to be symptom-free, you will repeat the reintroduce/observe cycle for that FODMAP for a total of 3 times.

You can use the same 21-day meal plan from the elimination phase but add in FODMAPs as you go. During this time, be sure to note how you feel before and after your meals. This will help you identify which FODMAPs are causing digestive problems. Use the charts on the following pages to help you figure out your next step and log your symptoms. Continue this pattern until you've tested every FODMAP (fructans, GOS, lactose, fructose, sorbitol, and mannitol).

REINTRODUCTION LOG

For recommended small, medium, and large serving sizes of foods other than those listed here, check the Monash University FODMAP Diet app, from the researchers who developed the FODMAP diet.

DAY	ACTION	SERVING SIZE	FODMAP	SYMPTOMS
1	Reintroduce	Small ex. ¼ cup milk or yogurt	Lactose	
2	Observe	-	Eat low-FODMAP only	
	If symptoms appear, continue to eat low-FODMAP for 3 days (or until symptoms disappear), then skip to GOS phase. If no symptoms, move onto medium serving.			
3	Reintroduce	Medium ex. ½ cup milk or yogurt	Lactose	
4	Observe	-	Eat low-FODMAP only	
	If symptoms appear, continue to eat low-FODMAP for 3 days (or until symptoms disappear), then skip to GOS phase. If no symptoms, move onto large serving.			
5	Reintroduce	Large ex. 1 cup milk or yogurt	Lactose	
6	Observe	-	Eat low-FODMAP only	
	If symptoms appear, continue to eat low-FODMAP for 3 days (or until symptoms disappear), then skip to GOS phase. If no symptoms, move onto GOS phase.			
7	Reintroduce	Small ex. ¼ cup canned black beans or 15 almonds	GOS	
8	Observe	-	Eat low-FODMAP only	
	If symptoms appear, continue to eat low-FODMAP for 3 days (or until symptoms disappear), then skip to fructans phase. If no symptoms, move onto medium serving.			

DAY	ACTION	SERVING SIZE	FODMAP	SYMPTOMS
9	Reintroduce	Medium ex. ⅓ cup canned black beans or 20 almonds	GOS	
10	Observe	-	Eat low-FODMAP only	
	If symptoms appear, continue to eat low-FODMAP for 3 days (or until symptoms disappear), then skip to fructans phase. If no symptoms, move onto large serving.			
11	Reintroduce	Large ex. ½ cup canned black beans or 25 almonds	GOS	
12	Observe	-	Eat low-FODMAP only	
	If symptoms appear, continue to eat to low-FODMAP for 3 days (or until symptoms disappear), then skip to fructans phase. If no symptoms, move onto fructans phase.			
13	Reintroduce	Small ex. ⅔ cup cooked wheat pasta or 1 slice of white wheat bread	Fructans	
14	Observe	-	Eat low-FODMAP only	
	If symptoms appear, continue to eat low-FODMAP for 3 days (or until symptoms disappear), then skip to fructose phase. If no symptoms, move onto medium serving.			
15	Reintroduce	Medium ex. 1 cup cooked wheat pasta or 2 slices of white wheat bread	Fructans	
16	Observe	-	Eat low-FODMAP only	
	If symptoms appear, continue to eat low-FODMAP for 3 days (or until symptoms disappear), then skip to fructose phase. If no symptoms, move onto a large serving.			

REINTRODUCTION LOG

DAY	ACTION	SERVING SIZE	FODMAP	SYMPTOMS
17	Reintroduce	Large ex. 1½ cups cooked wheat pasta or 3 slices of white wheat bread	Fructans	
18	Observe	-	Eat low-FODMAP only	
	If symptoms appear, continue to eat low-FODMAP for 3 days (or until symptoms disappear), then skip to fructose phase. If no symptoms, move onto fructose phase.			
19	Reintroduce	Small ex. 1 tsp honey or ¼ medium-sized mango	Fructose	
20	Observe	-	Eat low-FODMAP only	
	If symptoms appear, continue to eat low-FODMAP for 3 days (or until symptoms disappear), then skip to sorbitol phase. If no symptoms, move onto medium serving.			
21	Reintroduce	Medium ex. 1 Tbsp honey or ½ medium-sized mango	Fructose	
22	Observe	-	Eat low-FODMAP only	
	If symptoms appear, continue to eat low-FODMAP for 3 days (or until symptoms disappear), then skip to sorbitol phase. If no symptoms, move onto a large serving.			
23	Reintroduce	Large ex. 2 Tbsp honey or 1 medium-sized mango	Fructose	
24	Observe	-	Eat low-FODMAP only	
	If symptoms appear, continue to eat low-FODMAP for 3 days (or until symptoms disappear), then skip to sorbitol phase. If no symptoms, move onto sorbitol phase.			

DAY	ACTION	SERVING SIZE	FODMAP	SYMPTOMS
25	Reintroduce	Small ex. ¼ avocado or 5 blackberries	Sorbitol	
26	Observe	-	Eat low-FODMAP only	
	If symptoms appear, continue to eat low-FODMAP for 3 days (or until symptoms disappear), then skip to mannitol phase. If no symptoms, move onto medium serving.			
27	Reintroduce	Medium ex. ⅓ avocado or 8 blackberries	Sorbitol	
28	Observe	-	Eat low-FODMAP only	
	If symptoms appear, continue to eat low-FODMAP for 3 days (or until symptoms disappear), then skip to mannitol phase. If no symptoms, move onto a large serving.			
29	Reintroduce	Large ex. ½ avocado or 10 blackberries	Sorbitol	
30	Observe	-	Eat low-FODMAP only	
	If symptoms appear, continue to eat low-FODMAP for 3 days (or until symptoms disappear), then skip to mannitol phase. If no symptoms, move onto mannitol phase.			
31	Reintroduce	Small ex. ½ medium celery stalk or ¼ cup cauliflower	Mannitol	
32	Observe	-	Eat low-FODMAP only	
	If symptoms appear, continue to eat low-FODMAP for 3 days (or until symptoms disappear), then skip to personalization phase. If no symptoms, move onto medium serving.			

REINTRODUCTION LOG

DAY	ACTION	SERVING SIZE	FODMAP	SYMPTOMS
33	Reintroduce	Medium ex. 1 medium celery stalk or ⅓ cup cauliflower	Mannitol	
34	Observe	-	Eat low-FODMAP only	
	If symptoms appear, continue to eat low-FODMAP for 3 days (or until symptoms disappear), then skip to personalization phase. If no symptoms, move onto large serving.			
35	Reintroduce	Large ex. 1½ medium celery stalks or ½ cup cauliflower	Mannitol	
36	Observe	-	Eat low-FODMAP only	
	If symptoms appear, continue to eat low-FODMAP for 3 days (or until symptoms disappear), then skip to personalization phase. If no symptoms, move onto personalization phase.			

CHAPTER 6

The **Personalization** Phase

Congratulations! At this point, you should know exactly which FODMAPs (and what serving sizes) trigger symptoms for you, so you're ready to start the personalization phase. This isn't so much a phase as it is a new way of living. Now you can customize your everyday meals to focus on all the delicious foods that work in harmony with your body and exclude the FODMAPs you're sensitive to.

Easy Meals

Need a quick low-FODMAP meal? Try some of Mirkin's favorite recipes in the next few pages. Feel free to adjust the proteins based on your hunger levels and don't be afraid to get creative. This is about building a way of eating you can stick with for life — so make it about you!

Make sure to download the Monash app so you can quickly look up the FODMAP content of foods when you're not near your book. If you go off track and eat something high-FODMAP that you can't tolerate, you might have symptoms for 2 to 4 days.

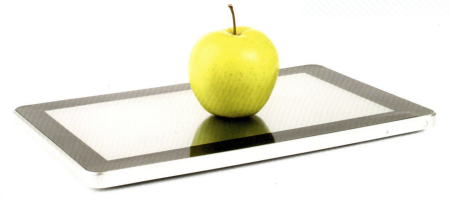

LOW-FODMAP BREAKFAST IDEAS

Egg and Vegetable Omelet

2 whole eggs plus 2 egg whites, ½ cup baby spinach, 1 cup chopped tomato, pinch of salt, and 1 oz shredded cheddar. Enjoy with 1 cup cantaloupe.

Cottage Cheese Power Breakfast

8 oz lactose-free cottage cheese combined with 1 cup strawberries, dash of cinnamon, and 2 Tbsp pecans.

Scrambled Eggs and Toast

1 whole egg and 3 egg whites scrambled in 1 tsp olive oil. Enjoy with 1 slice Udi's toast topped with 1 tsp Land-o-Lakes Light Butter with Canola Oil. 1 sliced orange.

Cinnamon Spice Oatmeal

1 cup steel-cut organic oatmeal cooked with 4 egg whites and topped with 2 Tbsp chopped walnuts, dash of cinnamon, dash of vanilla extract, and ½ cup strawberries.

Mexican-Style Eggs

In a medium skillet lightly coated with butter, scramble 2 whole eggs plus 2 egg whites with 1 Tbsp milk and a pinch of salt. Top cooked eggs with ½ oz low-fat shredded Cheddar cheese and 1 cup diced tomatoes. Serve with 2 corn tortilla sliders.

Cheese and Bacon Wrap

½ Food for Life Brown Rice Tortilla topped with ¼ cup shredded Mexican-style cheese, 2 slices nitrate-free turkey bacon, and 6 sliced cherry tomatoes.

Eggs and Bacon

In a medium skillet, cook 2 whole eggs in 1 tsp butter. Enjoy with 1 slice whole-grain Udi's toast, 2 slices extra-lean nitrate-free turkey bacon, and 1 cup cubed melon.

Cottage Cheese and Seed Butter

In a medium bowl, mix 6 oz lactose-free cottage cheese with 1 cup strawberries and 2 Tbsp sunflower seed butter.

Turkey Tacos

In a medium skillet lightly coated with butter, warm 2 corn tortilla sliders. Top each with ½ slice jack cheese and 1 oz warmed turkey deli slices. Top each with butter lettuce, chopped tomato, and 1½ tsp Best Foods Canola Mayonnaise. Enjoy with ½ cup strawberries and ½ cup lactose-free milk.

Easy Eggs

2 hard-boiled eggs with 1 slice whole-grain Udi's toast topped with 1 tsp light butter. Enjoy with ¼ cup lactose-free low-fat cottage cheese with ½ cup cubed melon.

LOW-FODMAP LUNCH IDEAS

Salmon Patty Wrap

3 oz cooked wild salmon wrapped in 1 large brown rice tortilla warmed on a skillet lightly coated with butter. Top with romaine lettuce, chopped tomato, scallion, and 2 Tbsp sour cream.

Shrimp Tacos

Heat 3 whole-grain corn tortilla sliders on a pan lightly coated with butter, and top each with 1½ Tbsp Mexican-style shredded cheese. At the same time, heat 4 oz raw frozen shrimp on a microwave-safe plate with 1 Tbsp water for 2 minutes on each side. Add shrimp to tortillas with chopped tomato, lettuce, and 1 Tbsp canola mayonnaise.

Open-Faced Turkey Sandwich with Cheese

1 slice Udi's whole-grain bread toasted and topped with 1 slice Cheddar (melted) and 3 oz turkey. Top with tomato, lettuce, and 1 Tbsp canola mayonnaise.

Shrimp and Pecan Salad

Large bowl of lettuce topped with 4 oz shrimp, 2 Tbsp toasted pecans, and 2 Tbsp low-FODMAP dressing.

Open-Faced Tuna Melt

1 slice Udi's whole-grain bread toasted and topped with 3 oz tuna salad mixed with 1 Tbsp canola mayonnaise and 1 slice melted Cheddar.

Grilled Chicken Salad with Roasted Bell Pepper

Large bed of mixed greens topped with 4 oz chicken breast, roasted red bell peppers, tomatoes, 2 Tbsp shredded Parmesan cheese, 1 Tbsp olive oil, and balsamic vinegar.

LOW-FODMAP LUNCH IDEAS

Tuna Wraps

Mix 3 oz tuna with 1 Tbsp canola mayonnaise, splash of lemon juice, ¼ celery stick, chopped, and ½ tsp fresh dill. Serve in large lettuce leaf with ½ cup melon on the side.

Grilled Steak Salad

In a large bowl, combine 3 oz cooked lean sirloin steak, 1 to 2 cups lettuce, ¼ cup grated carrots, ¼ cup cherry tomatoes, and ¼ cup sliced bell pepper slices. Drizzle 1 Tbsp red wine vinegar and 1 Tbsp olive oil on top.

Roasted Chicken and Vegetable Wrap

Heat 1 large brown rice tortilla on medium skillet lightly coated with butter. Top with 3 oz sliced cooked chicken breast, a few roasted carrots, zucchini, red pepper, and eggplant. Drizzle with ½ Tbsp balsamic vinegar and 1 oz crumbled goat cheese.

Tip: Prep a big batch of roasted vegetables on Sunday to make quick wraps and salads.

Niçoise Salad

In a large bowl, combine 1 to 2 cups lettuce, 3 oz tuna, 1 sliced hard-boiled egg, ⅓ cup cherry tomatoes, 2 Tbsp black olives, 1 Tbsp olive oil, salt, and pepper.

Open-Faced Caprese Sandwich

Top 1 slice toasted Udi's bread with 3 oz cooked and sliced chicken breast, 1 to 2 oz fresh mozzarella, 2 slices tomato, and 1 or 2 fresh basil leaves. Drizzle with ½ Tbsp olive oil and balsamic vinegar.

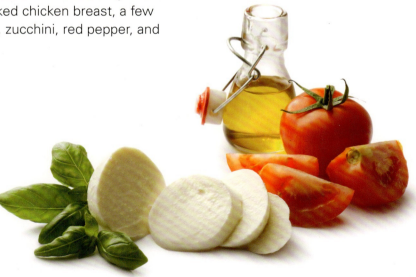

LOW-FODMAP DINNER IDEAS

Chicken and Strawberry Salad

Top a bed of butter lettuce and organic wild arugula with 6 oz of grilled chicken breast, sliced sweet baby bell pepper, organic strawberries, organic sweet cherry tomatoes, and 2 Tbsp avocado. Top with 1 Tbsp Fody Maple Dijon Dressing.

Grilled Salmon and Spinach

4 oz of grilled salmon topped with lemon, salt, and pepper. Enjoy with a 3-oz baked potato topped with 2 Tbsp sour cream and spinach sautéed in garlic-infused olive oil.

Shrimp and Veggie Skewers

Grill 6 oz shrimp on skewers with ½ red bell pepper, ½ summer squash, and 3 oz sliced potato coated with 1 Tbsp of garlic-infused oil and seasoned with a dash of salt and pepper.

Grilled Chicken Salad

6 oz grilled chicken tossed with mixed greens, strawberries, 2 Tbsp feta, and scallion. Drizzle with 2 tsp of garlic-infused olive oil and 1 Tbsp of balsamic or rice vinegar.

Sunflower Seed Crunch Salad

4 oz grilled chicken, 2 Tbsp Parmesan, sliced tomato, scallion, radish, 1 to 2 Tbsp sunflower seeds, and 2 Tbsp avocado over mixed greens with 1 Tbsp low-FODMAP dressing.

Shrimp Stir-Fry

6 oz shrimp, ½ cup broccoli, ½ small carrot, dash of scallion, ½ yellow squash, ½ red bell pepper, and ½ cup water chestnuts sautéed in 1½ tsp garlic-infused oil, fresh ginger, and low-sodium soy sauce over ½ cup rice.

Turkey Burger

4 oz turkey burger over bed of greens, 2 Tbsp avocado, and tomato topped with 2 Tbsp Parmesan and 2 Tbsp low-FODMAP dressing.

Scallops and Greens

6 large cooked scallops over mixed greens with a 3-oz baked potato topped with 2 Tbsp sour cream.

Add Some Flavor!

Try incorporating these low-FODMAP ingredients to your favorite recipes for a flavor boost:

Basil	Curry powder
Capers	Mustard
Chili powder	Oregano
Cilantro	Paprika
Cinnamon	Soy sauce

3 oz sliced turkey wrapped in lettuce leaves with 1 tsp olive oil mayo, Dijon mustard, and ½ cup baby tomatoes.

1 sprouted corn tortilla topped with 2 oz shrimp, fresh tomatoes, and 1½ Tbsp shredded Cheddar.

1 3-oz pouch tuna fish with Dijon mustard, 6 Mary's Gone Crackers, and ½ cup baby tomatoes.

½ cup lactose-free cottage cheese, ¼ cup blueberries, and ½ cup strawberries.

1 stick string cheese with 6 baby bell peppers and ⅓ cup baby carrots.

1 slice whole-grain Udi's toast topped with 2 oz turkey breast, lettuce, tomato, and mustard.

1 stick string cheese wrapped with 1 oz turkey in lettuce leaves with mustard alongside ⅓ cup baby carrots.

3 oz cooked chicken breast with Dijon mustard, baby tomatoes, and ⅓ cup baby carrots.

1 oz Cheddar with 6 whole-grain crackers and ½ cup baby bell peppers.

6 oz plain 0% fat Greek yogurt (be sure to take a Lactaid supplement before eating if sensitive to lactose) with 1 tsp sunflower seed butter, 1 tsp toasted pecan pieces, and ½ cup strawberries.

2 hard-boiled eggs with 6 cherry tomatoes.

½ cup baby carrots with 1 Tbsp sunflower seed butter.

1 Tbsp peanut butter with 1 square dark chocolate (over 85% cocoa).

2 Tbsp ricotta cheese mixed with ½ cup heated strawberries, 1 Tbsp toasted pecan pieces, and dash cinnamon.

Lettuce leaves filled with 2 oz turkey, 2 Tbsp whipped cream cheese, and scallion tips.

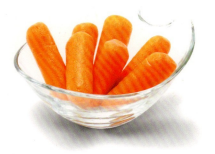

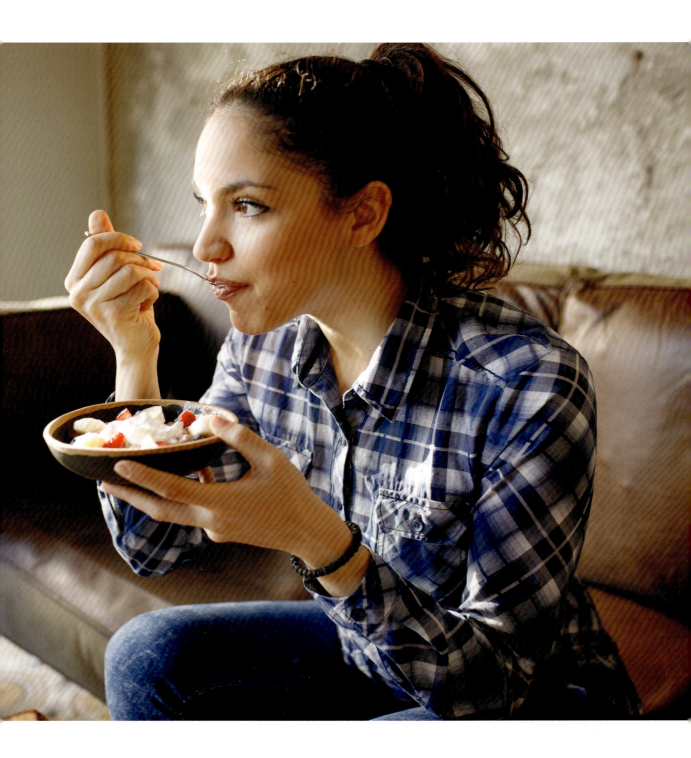

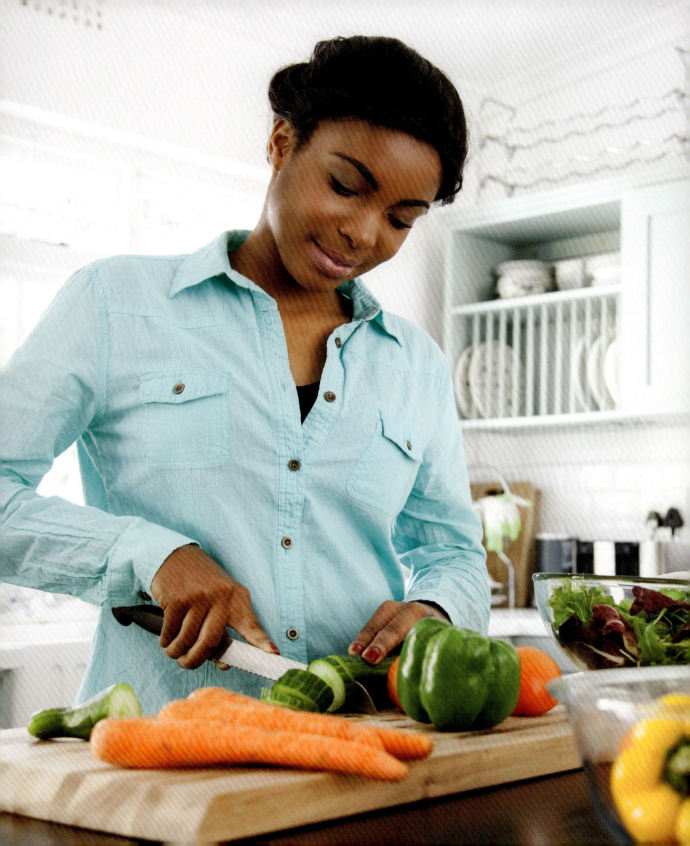

CHAPTER 7

Low-FODMAP Recipes

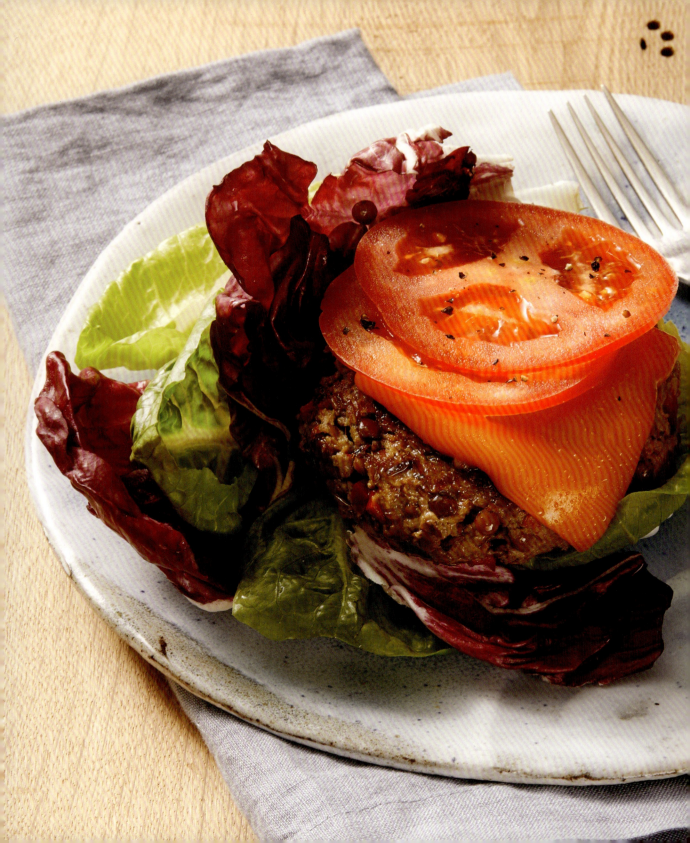

Lentil and Beef Burgers in Lettuce Wraps

ACTIVE 12 MIN. | TOTAL 22 MIN. | SERVES 2

1 In a medium bowl, mash the lentils.

2 In a large bowl, mix mashed lentils, bell pepper, scallions, ground beef, salt, and pepper. Form into 2 patties.

3 Spray a large skillet with avocado oil spray. Heat pan over medium-high, and add patties. Sear until dark brown on one side, about 5 minutes, then flip patties and repeat on other side. Lay cheese on patties after flipping them.

4 Serve in lettuce leaves with sliced tomato and avocado.

NUTRITION (per serving): 324 cal, 27 g pro, 21 g carb, 8.5 g fiber, 4 g sugars (0 g added sugars), 15 g fat (6.5 g sat fat), 62 mg chol, 227 mg sodium

¾ cup canned lentils, rinsed

¼ cup finely chopped red bell pepper

⅛ cup finely chopped scallions

¼ lb extra-lean ground beef (97% lean)

Salt and pepper, to taste

Avocado oil spray

2 1-oz slices Cheddar cheese

Large lettuce leaves (iceberg or romaine)

2 small vine-ripe or Campari tomatoes, sliced

¼ avocado, sliced into 4 pieces

High-Protein Oatmeal

½ cup old-fashioned oats

½ tsp cinnamon

Dash of pure vanilla extract

Pinch of sea salt

1 cup lactose-free milk

¼ cup egg whites

½ cup strawberries (frozen or fresh)

1 Tbsp chia seeds

1 In a medium saucepan over medium-high, combine oats, cinnamon, vanilla extract, sea salt, and milk, stirring occasionally. Cook until all the liquid has been absorbed, 6 to 7 minutes.

2 Add egg whites and strawberries to oats and stir constantly so egg whites don't form a scramble. They should turn into a thick, fluffy consistency after approximately 1 to 2 minutes.

3 Once all liquid is absorbed and oatmeal is cooked through, place in small bowl, add chia seeds, and enjoy!

NUTRITION (per serving): 350 cal, 23 g pro, 50 g carb, 10 g fiber, 16 g sugars (0 g added sugars), 8 g fat (1 g sat fat), 5 mg chol, 227 mg sodium

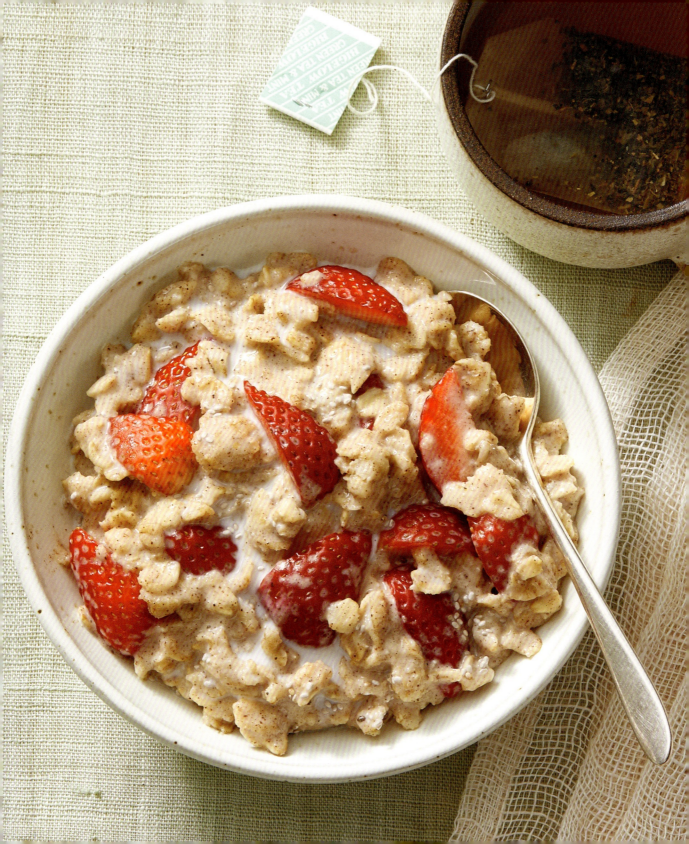

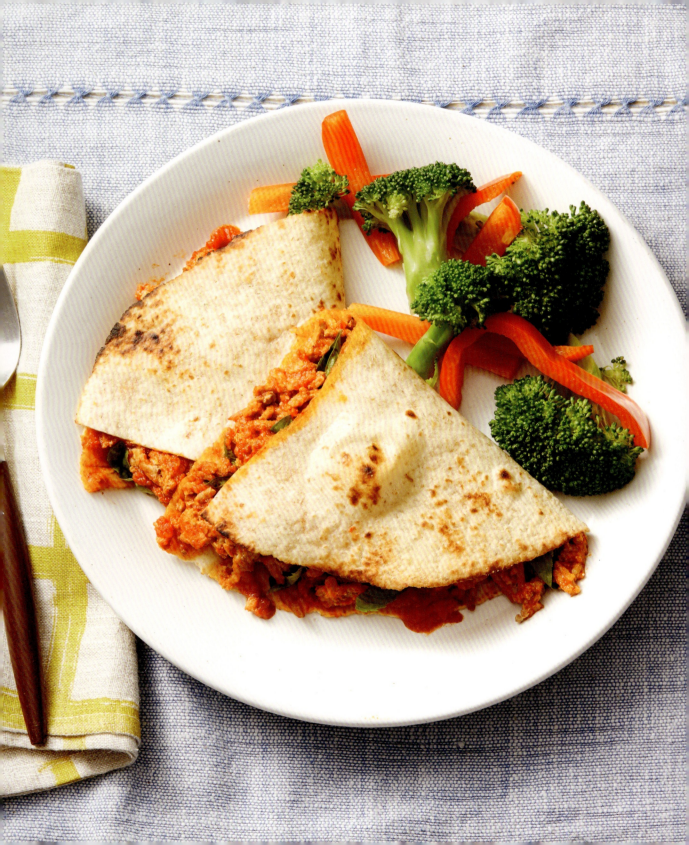

Ground Turkey Calzone

ACTIVE 15 MIN. | TOTAL 15 MIN. | SERVES 2

1 In a medium nonstick skillet over medium-high heat, cook the ground turkey. Stir and crumble with a spatula until lightly browned, 6 to 7 minutes.

2 Meanwhile, steam the broccoli and bell pepper in a microwave–safe dish with 2 Tbsp of water, for approximately 5 minutes or steam in a steamer basket for 5 to 8 minutes, or until desired tenderness.

3 After ground turkey is browned, add marinara sauce and fresh basil to a large skillet and simmer for 2 to 3 minutes.

4 Coat a second medium skillet with avocado oil spray and heat on medium-high. Add tortillas one at a time, and cook until lightly browned, approximately 45 seconds per side.

5 As you remove each tortilla from the skillet, add turkey mixture with some Parmesan to the tortilla and wrap it up.

6 Serve with steamed veggies.

½ lb extra-lean ground turkey breast

1½ cups chopped broccoli

½ red bell pepper, sliced

2 medium brown rice tortillas

1 cup Low-FODMAP marinara sauce (p. 102)

Fresh basil, julienned

2 Tbsp grated Parmesan cheese

Avocado oil spray

NUTRITION (per serving): 400 cal, 35 g pro, 45 g carb, 8 g fiber, 11 g sugars (0g added sugars), 8 g fat (2 g sat fat), 69 mg chol, 450 mg sodium

Pork Chops

1 Heat oven to 475°F. In a medium oven-safe dish, place pork chops. Coat with olive oil and vinegar.

2 Top with ground almonds, tomatoes, and bell pepper. Bake for approximately 40 minutes, until it smells delicious!

NUTRITION (per serving): 380 cal, 41 g pro, 12 g carb, 4 g fiber, 6 g sugars (0 g added sugars), 19 g fat (1 g sat fat), 117 mg chol, 110 mg sodium

12-oz pork chop (with bone)

1 Tbsp extra virgin olive oil

2 Tbsp balsamic vinegar

15 almonds, ground

2 small tomatoes, sliced

1 cup sliced green bell pepper

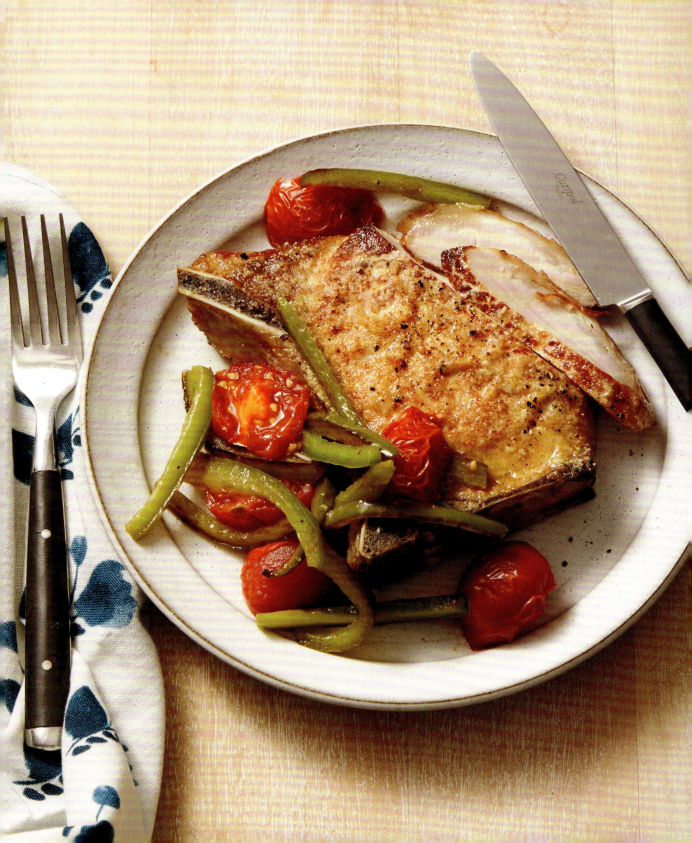

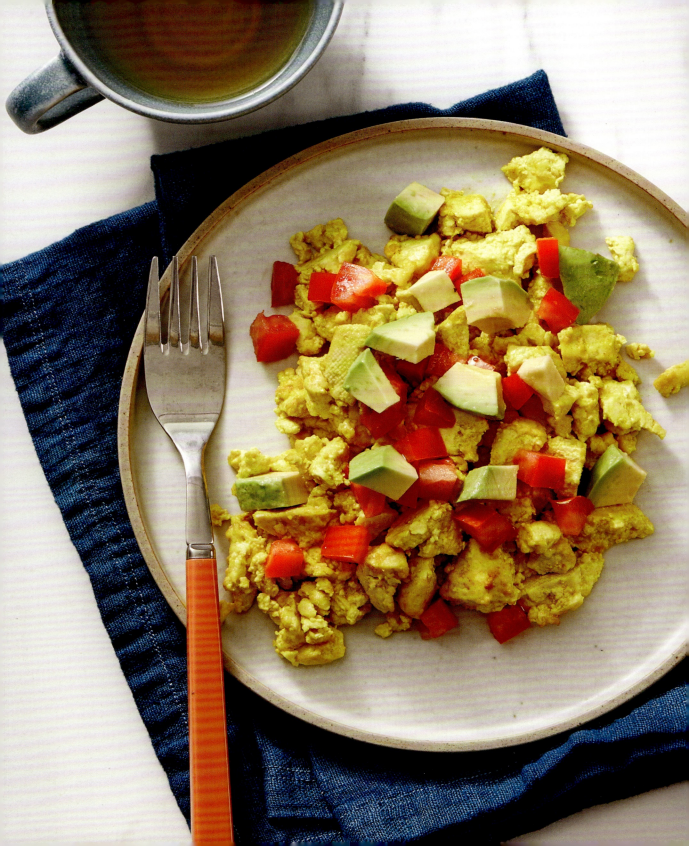

Tofu Scramble with Diced Tomato and Avocado

ACTIVE 15 MIN. | TOTAL 15 MIN. | SERVES 1

1 In a large skillet over medium, heat olive oil. Add tofu and mash with spatula.

2 Cook, stirring frequently, until water from tofu has evaporated, 3 to 4 minutes.

3 Add nutritional yeast, dash of salt, and turmeric. Cook and stir for approximately 5 minutes.

4 Pour milk into skillet and stir to combine.

5 When milk is absorbed, serve with chopped tomato and small avocado cubes.

NUTRITION (per serving): 355 cal, 31 g pro, 19 g carb, 10 g fiber, 5.5 g sugars (0 g added sugars), 19 g fat (2.5 g sat fat), 0 mg chol, 77 mg sodium

½ tsp garlic-infused olive oil

½ 16-oz block firm tofu

1 Tbsp nutritional yeast

Salt

⅛ tsp turmeric

1 Tbsp lactose-free, fat-free milk

1 medium vine-ripe tomato, chopped

2 Tbsp avocado, cubed

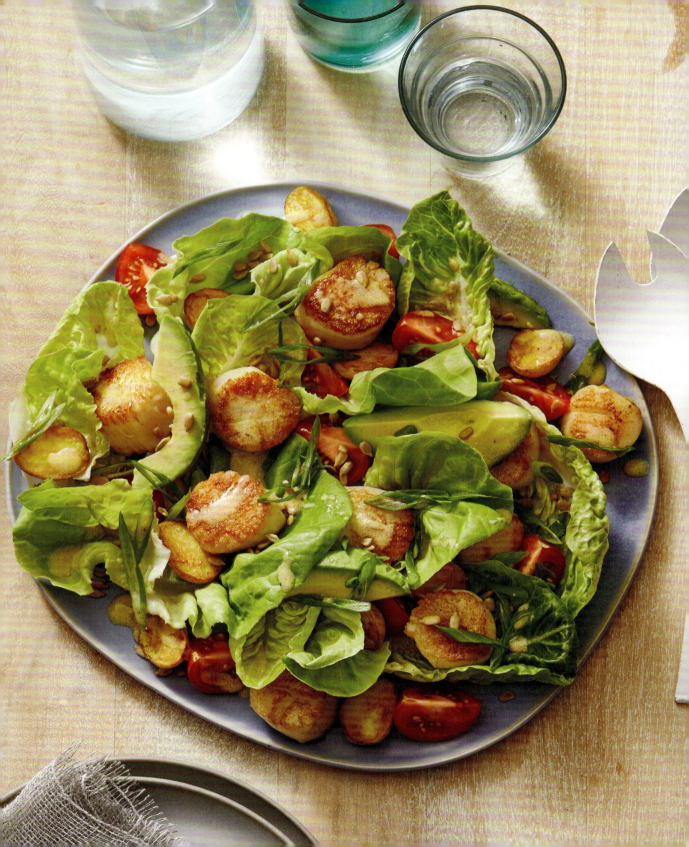

Scallop Salad

1 If scallops are frozen, defrost them in microwave or in refrigerator in sealed bag in water.

2 Heat a large skillet on medium-high, and coat very lightly with avocado oil spray.

3 Remove scallops from microwave or bag, dry them well, and then add them to prepared skillet with dash of salt and pepper. Flip them after 2 to 3 minutes.

4 Meanwhile, place washed, pierced potato in microwave and cook on high for 5 minutes.

5 In a large bowl, mix together the lettuces, tomatoes, and avocado.

6 Remove potato from microwave and slice like thick potato chips. Add potato slices and dash of salt to scallops in skillet over medium-high heat. Cook potatoes on each side until lightly browned, about 1 minute per side.

7 Once scallops and potatoes are cooked, add to salad. Top salad with remaining ingredients. Mix everything together and enjoy!

NUTRITION (per serving): 360 cal, 20 g pro, 22 g carb, 7 g fiber, 4 g sugars (0 g added sugars), 25 g fat (3 g sat fat), 27 mg chol, 510 mg sodium

½ lb fresh or frozen scallops

Avocado oil spray

Dash of salt and pepper

1 small white potato

4 cups baby romaine lettuce

4 cups butter lettuce

2 medium Campari or vine-ripe tomatoes, sliced

½ avocado (split into 4 parts)

4 scallions, chopped (green parts only)

2 Tbsp sunflower seeds

2 Tbsp low-FODMAP dressing (or use recipe on p. 104)

Protein Pasta

ACTIVE 10 MIN. | TOTAL 20 MIN. | SERVES 2

1 Cook pasta according to pkg. directions.

2 Heat a medium skillet on medium-high, and coat lightly with avocado oil spray.

3 Cook ground chicken, chopping it and stirring until it lightly browns, about 6 to 7 minutes.

4 In a separate large skillet, heat garlic-infused oil over medium heat, add vegetables, and cook approximately 5 minutes, or until desired tenderness.

5 Combine vegetables and chicken in large skillet and add marinara sauce. Heat until it simmers, 5 minutes.

6 Top with Parmesan cheese.

NUTRITION (per serving): 400 cal, 28 g pro, 40 g carb, 10 g fiber, 9 g sugars (0 g added sugars), 15 g fat (4 g sat fat), 60 mg chol, 580 mg sodium

1 oz chickpea pasta (1 cup cooked)

Avocado oil spray

4 oz ground chicken

2 tsp garlic-infused oil

1 cup chopped broccoli heads

1 yellow squash, thinly sliced

1 cup eggplant, thinly sliced

2 cups baby spinach

¼ cup chopped scallion

1 cup Low-FODMAP Marinara Sauce (p. 102), or 2 cups Fody brand sauce

2 Tbsp grated Parmesan cheese

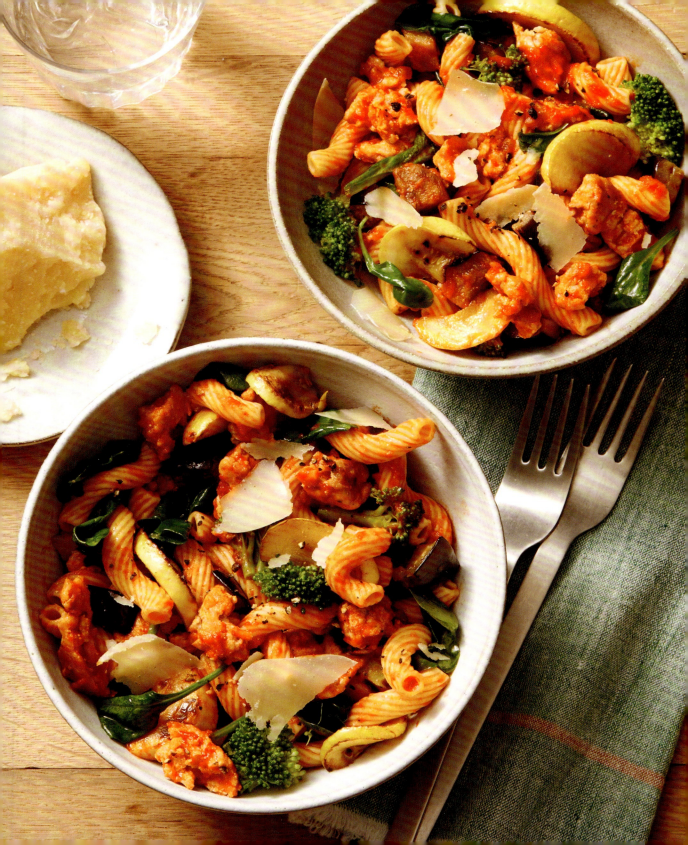

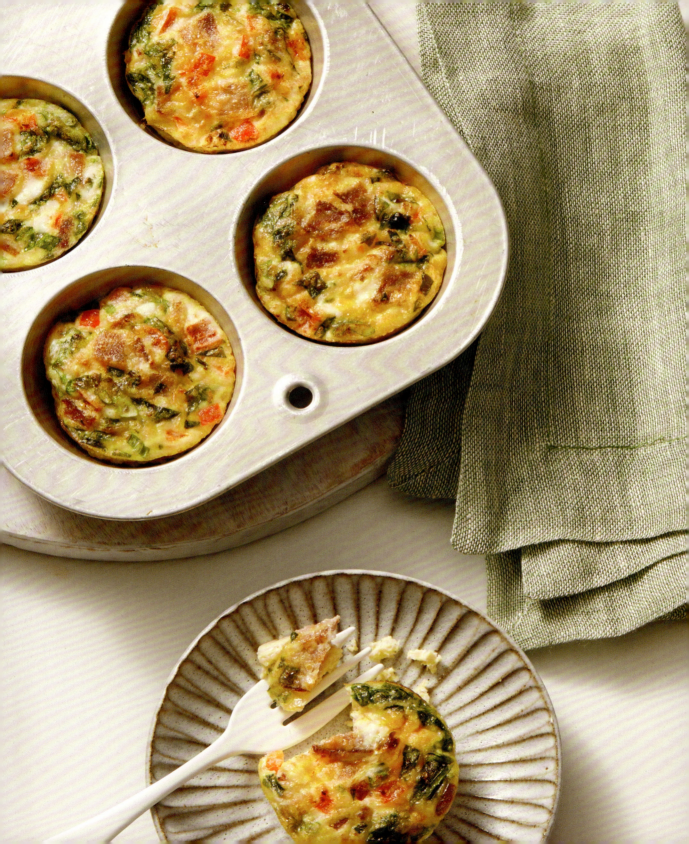

Egg Muffins

ACTIVE 5 MIN. | TOTAL 30 MIN. | SERVES 3 (2-MUFFIN SERVING)

1 Heat oven to 350°F. Spray a muffin tin with cooking spray.

2 In a large bowl, whisk eggs and egg whites and season with salt and pepper. Mix in the remaining ingredients.

3 Fill each muffin cup and place tins on a cookie sheet. Bake 20 to 25 minutes, or until set.

NUTRITION (per serving): 165 cal, 14 g pro, 2.5 g carb, 2 g fiber, 2 g sugars (0 g added sugars), 11 g fat (6 g sat fat), 290 mg chol, 267 mg sodium

Avocado oil cooking spray

5 large eggs

1 cup egg whites

¼ tsp kosher salt

Black pepper

3 strips cooked organic turkey bacon, chopped

3 Tbsp thawed frozen spinach, drained

3 Tbsp diced tomatoes

3 Tbsp diced scallions (green part only)

3 Tbsp diced bell pepper

2 oz shredded Cheddar cheese

Salmon Parmesan with Broccoli and Potato

ACTIVE 10 MIN. | TOTAL 20 MIN. | SERVES 2

1 Heat oven to 400°F. Line a baking sheet with foil.

2 In a small bowl, whisk together the mayo and cheese.

3 Place fish on prepared baking sheet. Cover fish with mayo mixture. Bake until fish flakes easily with fork, 12 to 15 minutes.

4 Meanwhile, steam the broccoli and bell pepper in a microwaveable dish with 2 Tbsp water for approximately 5 minutes or steam in a steamer basket for 5 to 8 minutes, or until desired tenderness.

5 Place the potatoes in a microwaveable dish and microwave on high for 5 minutes.

6 Heat a large skillet coated lightly with avocado oil over medium-high heat.

7 Slice the potatoes and add them to the hot skillet with a dash of salt and pepper (if desired), and cook for approximately 2 minutes per side, or until lightly browned.

8 Serve everything together. Enjoy!

NUTRITION (per serving): 360 cal, 33 g pro, 20 g carb, 4 g fiber, 3.5 g sugars (0 g added sugars), 16 g fat (2.5 g sat fat), 80 mg chol, 300 mg sodium

2 Tbsp olive oil mayonnaise

1 Tbsp grated Parmesan cheese

2 skinless wild salmon fillets (½ lb)

1½ cups broccoli head pieces

1 red bell pepper, sliced

2 extra-small white potatoes

1 tsp avocado oil

Dash of salt and pepper, to taste

TIP
Try a little low-FODMAP ketchup on the potato!

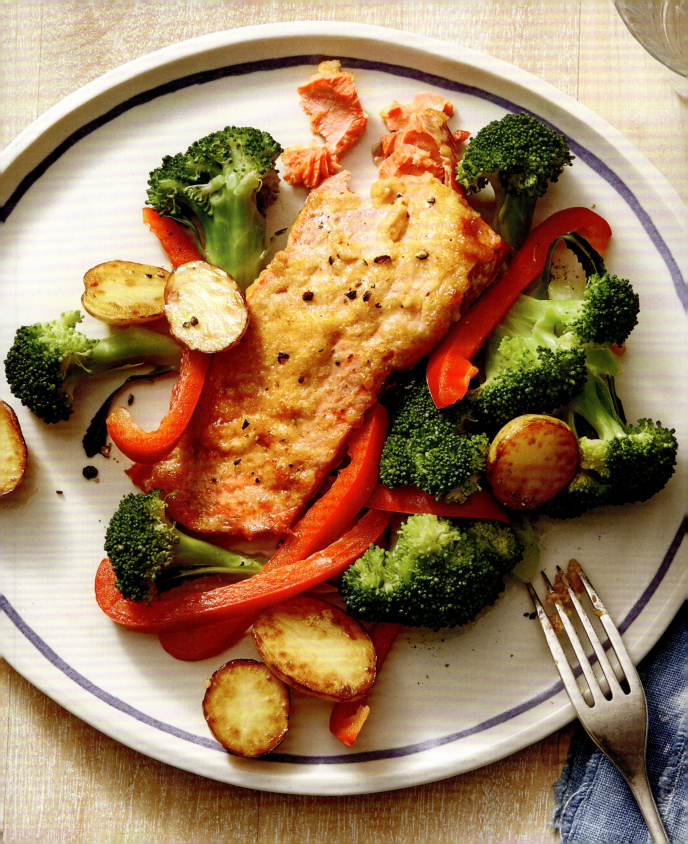

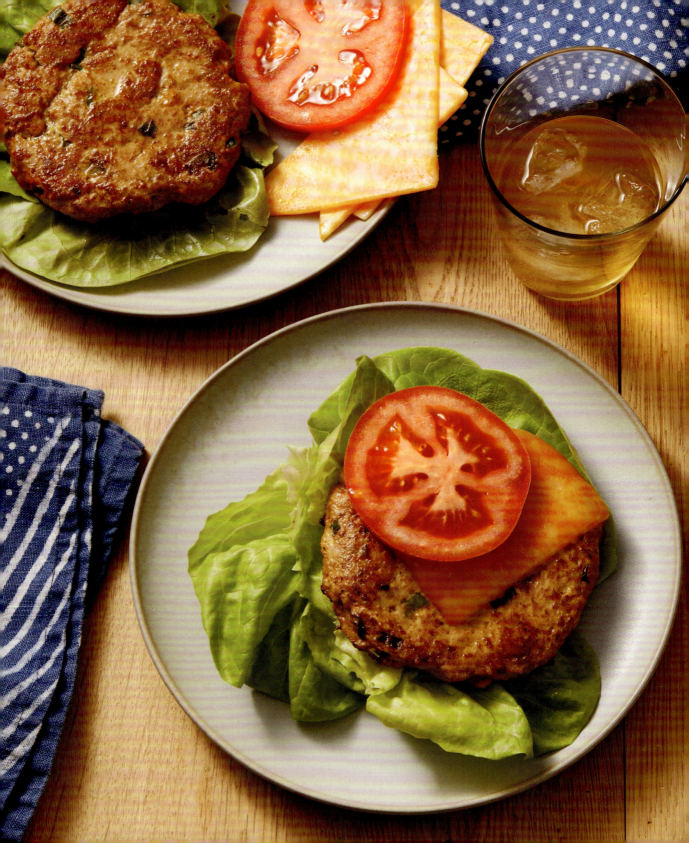

Sarah's Turkey Burger

1 In a large bowl, combine turkey, egg, egg whites, Parmesan, scallions, and soy sauce. Form 4 patties approximately 1½ in. thick.

2 Spray a large skillet on medium-high with avocado oil cooking spray. Once skillet is hot, add the patties and cook for about 5 to 6 minutes on each side.

3 When patties are finished cooking, top with cheese and allow to melt slightly. Remove patties from skillet and place on lettuce leaves.

4 Top with tomato and wrap it up!

NUTRITION (per serving): 360 cal, 35 g pro, 7 g carb, 2 g fiber, 3 g sugars (0 g added sugars), 21.5 g fat (9 g sat fat), 155 mg chol, 600 mg sodium

1 lb ground turkey (93% lean)

1 large egg

2 large egg whites

¼ cup grated Parmesan cheese

¼ cup chopped scallions (green parts only)

¼ cup reduced-sodium soy sauce

Avocado oil cooking spray

Iceberg lettuce or large romaine lettuce leaves

4 1-oz slices Colby jack cheese

2 medium Campari or vine-ripe tomatoes, sliced

Caesar Chicken Wraps

ACTIVE 5 MIN. | TOTAL 30 MIN. | SERVES 4

1 Heat the oven to 400°F. Lightly grease a baking dish with avocado oil.

2 In a medium bowl, toss chicken breasts with oil, salt, and pepper.

3 Bake chicken breasts 22 to 26 minutes, or until they reach 165°F. Let them cool slightly before slicing.

4 Pull lettuce apart to create individual wraps. Top with chicken, cherry tomatoes, and Parmesan cheese.

5 Drizzle Caesar dressing on each wrap.

NUTRITION (per serving): 330 cal, 37 g pro, 7.5 g carb, 4 g fiber, 3 g sugars (0 g added sugars), 17 g fat (3 g sat fat), 110 mg chol, 240 mg sodium

1 tsp avocado oil

1 lb boneless, skinless chicken breast

1 Tbsp garlic-infused olive oil

Salt and pepper, to taste

1 head romaine lettuce or iceberg lettuce

1½ cups cherry tomatoes, sliced

¼ cup grated Parmesan cheese

⅓ cup low-FODMAP Caesar dressing

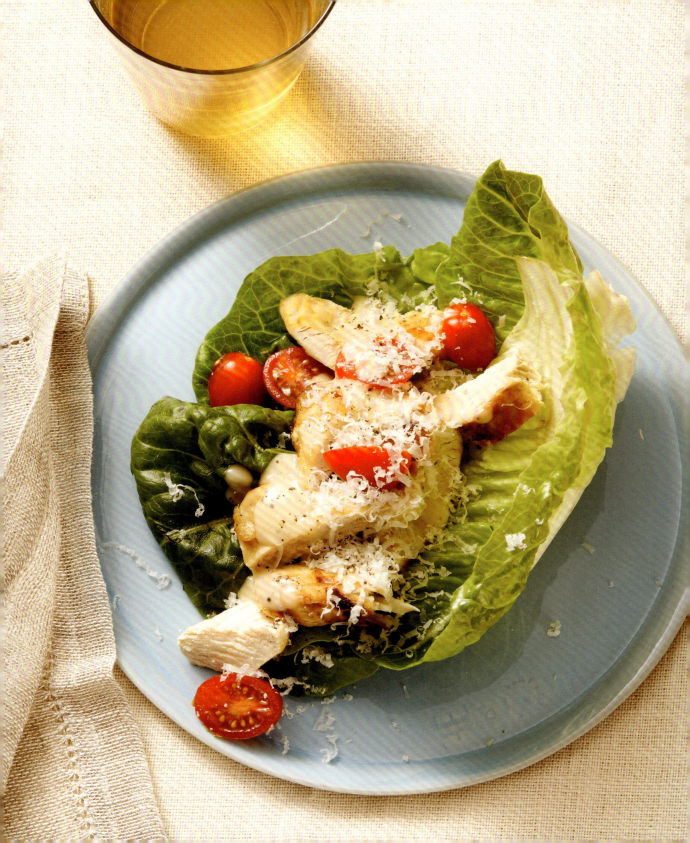

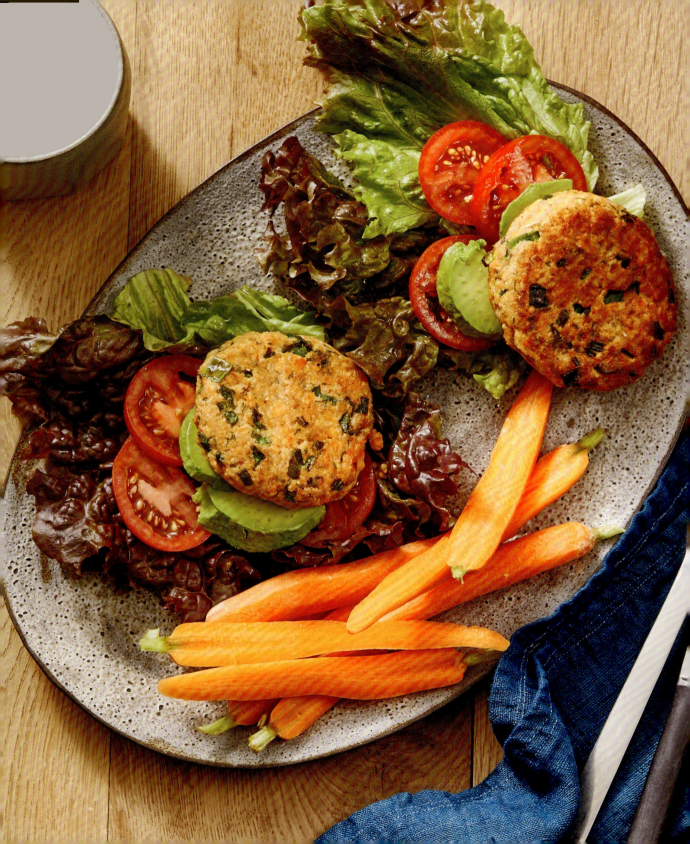

Salmon Burgers

1 In a large bowl, mix together salmon (allow salmon to sit out for 10 minutes if refrigerated), lemon zest, scallions, dill, mustard, salt, pepper, egg, and Parmesan. Form 3 to 4 patties.

2 In a large skillet over medium-high, heat oil. Once oil is hot, place burger patties in pan and cook until cooked through and lightly browned, 5 to 6 minutes on each side.

3 Top with sliced avocado and sliced tomato and place in lettuce leaves. Serve with baby carrots.

NUTRITION (per serving): 350 cal, 35 g pro, 11 g carb, 7 g fiber, 4 g sugars (0 g added sugars), 19 g fat (4 g sat fat), 4 mg chol, 340 mg sodium

6 oz wild-caught salmon, baked and chopped (or canned wild salmon, well drained)

¼ tsp lemon zest

4 scallions, chopped (green part only)

½ Tbsp chopped fresh dill

1 tsp Dijon mustard

⅛ tsp salt

⅛ tsp pepper

1 large egg

⅛ cup grated Parmesan cheese

1 Tbsp avocado oil

½ avocado, sliced into 8 equal pieces

2 medium vine-ripe tomatoes, sliced

Large lettuce leaves

1½ cups baby carrots

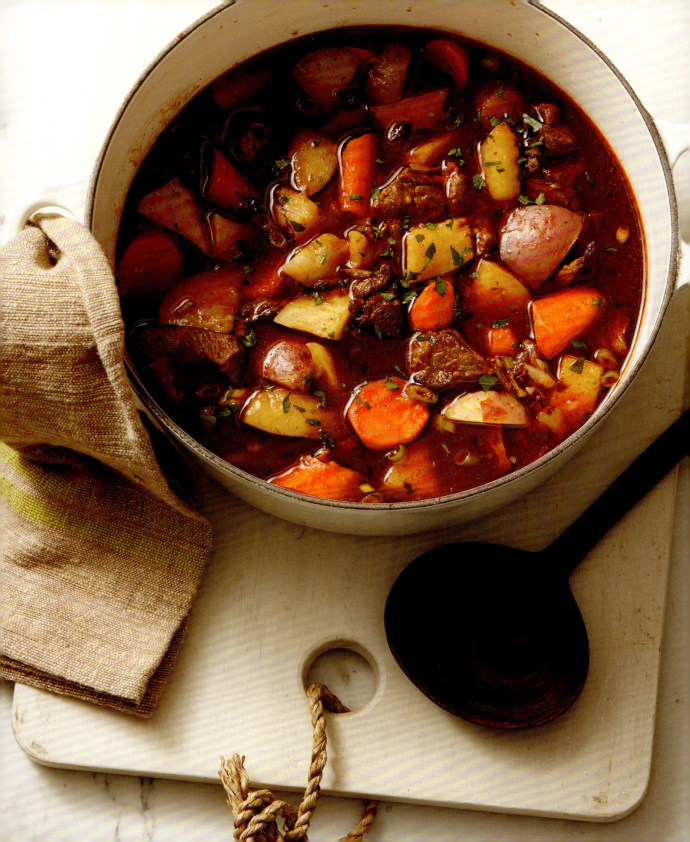

Beef Stew

ACTIVE 15 MIN. | TOTAL 3 HR. 15 MIN. | SERVES 2

1 In a large skillet over medium-high, sauté scallion in oil.

2 Add beef and brown well on all sides.

3 Add tomato paste, bay leaf, salt, pepper, and enough water to cover meat. Mix well. Bring to a boil, then cover and simmer for 2 hours.

4 Add carrots, potatoes, and more water, if required. Cover and simmer until carrots, potatoes, and meat are tender.

5 Finally, add chopped parsley and serve.

NUTRITION (per serving): 380 cal, 36 g pro, 26 g carb, 5 g fiber, 4.5 g sugars (0 g added sugars), 15 g fat (4.5 g sat fat), 98 mg chol, 127 mg sodium

1 Tbsp sliced scallion

1½ tsp garlic-infused olive oil

1 lb sirloin steak, trimmed and cubed

1 Tbsp tomato paste

1 bay leaf

Salt and pepper, to taste

1 large carrot, cut into chunks

1 9-oz potato, cut in 8 pieces

Chopped parsley, to taste

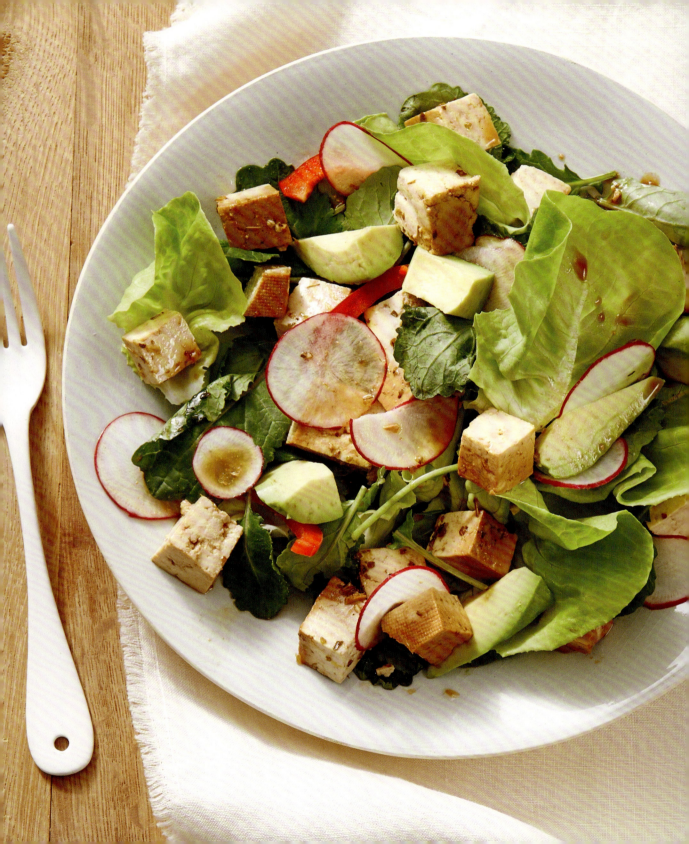

Marinated Tofu Salad

1 In a large bowl, combine soy sauce, oil, vinegar, brown sugar, lemon zest, and oregano.

2 Add tofu cubes and toss until all sides are well coated.

3 Marinate for 30 minutes or overnight in fridge.

4 In a separate bowl, mix power greens, avocado, bell pepper, and radish.

5 Toss with tofu and low-FODMAP dressing.

NUTRITION (per serving): 400 cal, 28 g pro, 12 g carb, 6 g fiber, 4.5 g sugars (4 g added sugars), 24 g fat (2 g sat fat), 0 mg chol, 425 mg sodium

¾ cup reduced-sodium soy sauce

½ Tbsp garlic-infused olive oil

1 Tbsp balsamic vinegar

1 tsp brown sugar, packed

½ tsp lemon zest

½ tsp oregano leaves

5 oz extra-firm tofu, drained and patted dry, cut into 1-in. cubes

4 cups power greens, including baby kale, baby spinach, chard, and mizuna

¼ avocado, chopped

½ red bell pepper, sliced

1 radish, sliced

2 Tbsp low-FODMAP dressing (or use recipe on p. 104)

Pecan-Crusted Salmon Salad

1 On a plate, lightly sprinkle salmon with salt and pepper. Coat both sides with Dijon mustard. Spread pecans over mustard on both sides.

2 In a large skillet over medium heat, coat pan with oil. Once hot, add salmon and cook until golden brown, about 3 to 4 minutes per side.

3 In a large bowl, mix all remaining ingredients, add salmon, and enjoy!

NUTRITION (per serving): 400 cal, 34 g pro, 15 g carb, 7 g fiber, 6 g sugars (0 g added sugars), 24 g fat (3 g sat fat), 78 mg chol, 275 mg sodium

5 oz wild salmon, at room temp

Dash kosher salt

Dash black pepper

½ Tbsp Dijon mustard

1 Tbsp crushed pecans

¾ tsp avocado oil

1 cup baby spinach

1 cup arugula

5 cherry tomatoes

2 Tbsp avocado, sliced

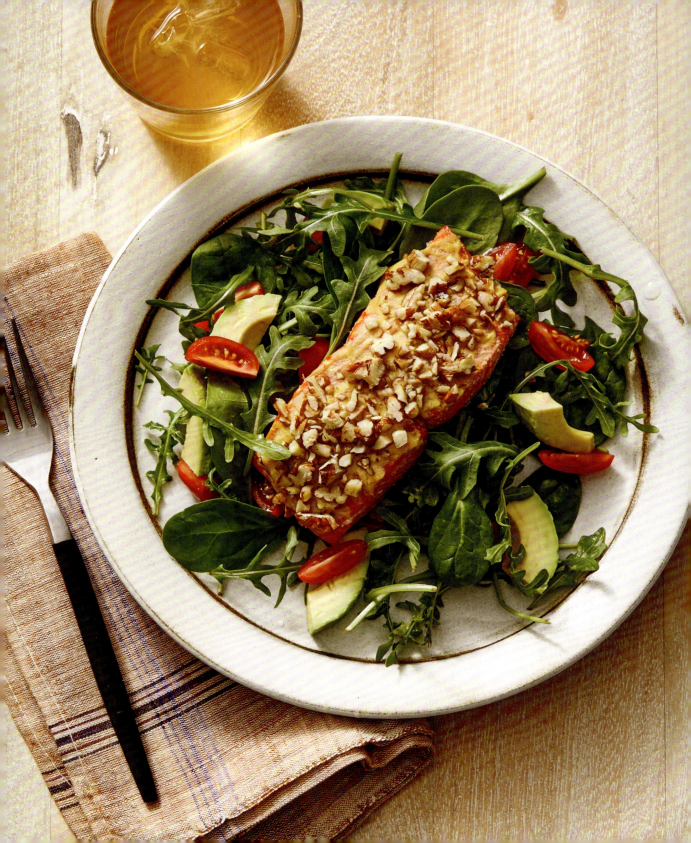

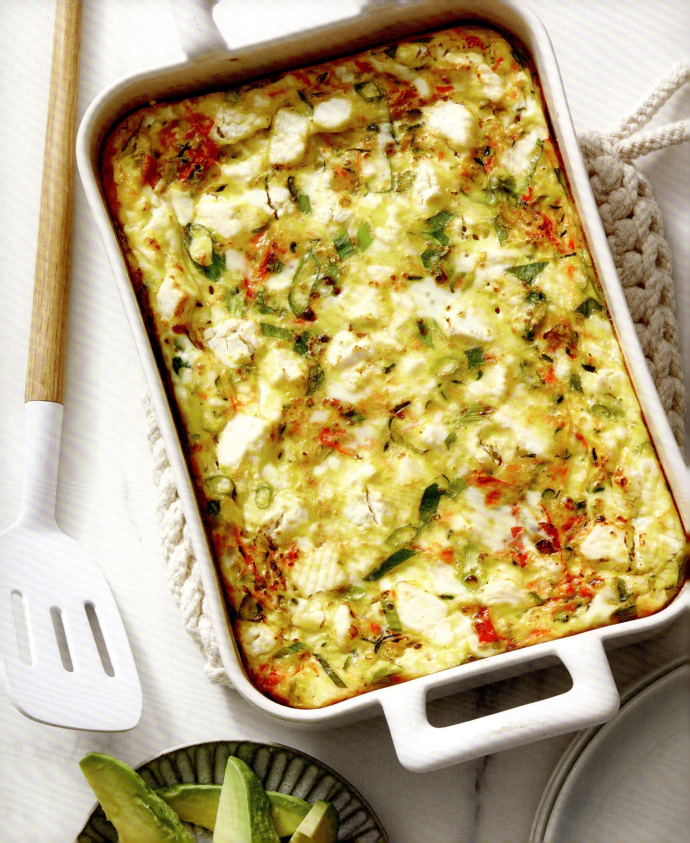

Zucchini, Bell Pepper, and Feta Frittata

ACTIVE 15 MIN. | TOTAL 50 MIN. | SERVES 4

1 Heat the oven to 350°F. Coat a 2-qt ovenproof dish (11- by 7-in.) with oil.

2 Into a medium bowl, grate the zucchini and bell pepper and season well with salt and pepper.

3 Lightly coat a large skillet with oil and heat it on medium-high. Add zucchini and bell pepper and cook until the vegetables are softened, 5 to 7 minutes. Using a wooden spoon, press vegetables against skillet side to squeeze out any excess liquid, then remove them from the skillet. Allow to cool for a few minutes.

4 In a large bowl, whisk together eggs, egg whites, milk, ¾ cup feta, scallion, and dash of salt and pepper.

5 Scoop vegetable mixture into oven dish and pour egg mixture on top. Crumble the remaining ¼ cup feta over top.

6 Bake until just set, 30 to 35 minutes.

NUTRITION (per serving): 210 cal, 20 g pro, 6 g carb, 4 g fiber, 5 g sugars (0 g added sugars), 11 g fat (5 g sat fat), 250 mg chol, 370 mg sodium

1 tsp garlic-infused olive oil

2 medium zucchinis

2 red bell peppers

Sea salt and pepper

6 medium eggs

1 cup liquid egg whites

¼ cup lactose-free milk

1 cup feta cheese, divided

¼ cup finely chopped scallion (green parts only)

TIP
This makes a great snack or side dish. Top with sour cream for a low-calorie burst of flavor.

Italian Turkey Meatloaf with Arugula Salad

ACTIVE 5 MIN. | TOTAL 45 MIN. | SERVES 4

1 Heat oven to 400°F.

2 In a large bowl, thoroughly combine turkey, Parmesan, marinara sauce, scallions, egg, and egg whites. Form a loaf with mixture and add to 2-qt baking dish (11- by 7-in.).

3 Bake until juices are clear, approximately 40 minutes.

4 While meatloaf is baking, prepare arugula salad. In a large bowl, top arugula with tomatoes, cucumber, and avocado. Split evenly among 4 plates.

5 In a small bowl, whisk together oil and vinegar and pour over each salad.

NUTRITION (per serving): 400 cal, 33 g pro, 18 g carb, 5 g fiber, 4.5 g sugars (0 g added sugars), 23 g fat (6 g sat fat), 130 mg chol, 330 mg sodium

1 lb ground turkey (93% lean)

½ cup Parmesan cheese

1 cup Low-FODMAP Marinara Sauce (p. 102)

⅓ cup chopped scallions (green parts only)

1 large egg

2 egg whites

8 cups arugula

4 tomatoes, sliced

1 cup sliced cucumber

½ avocado, sliced

4 tsp olive oil

2 Tbsp balsamic vinegar

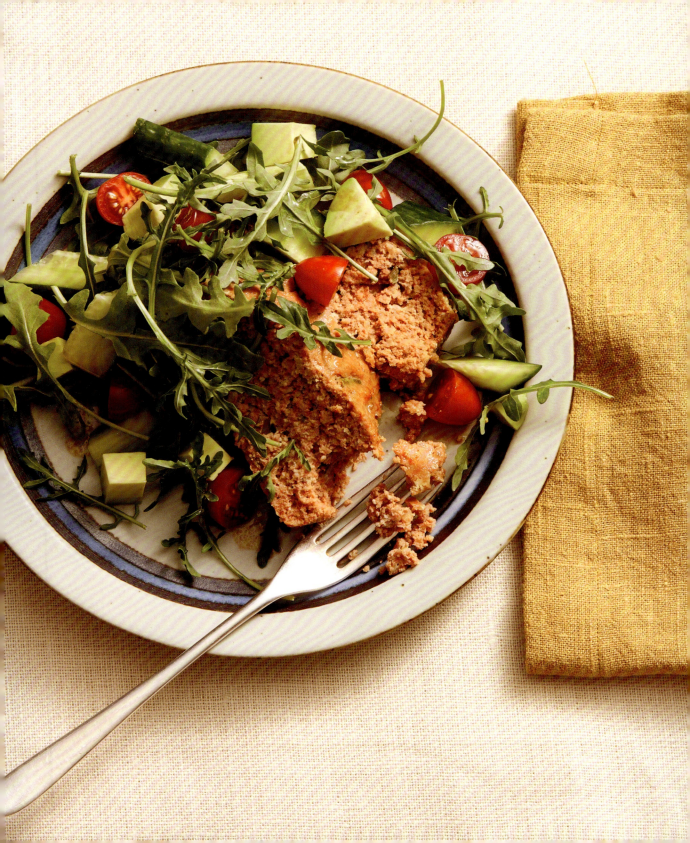

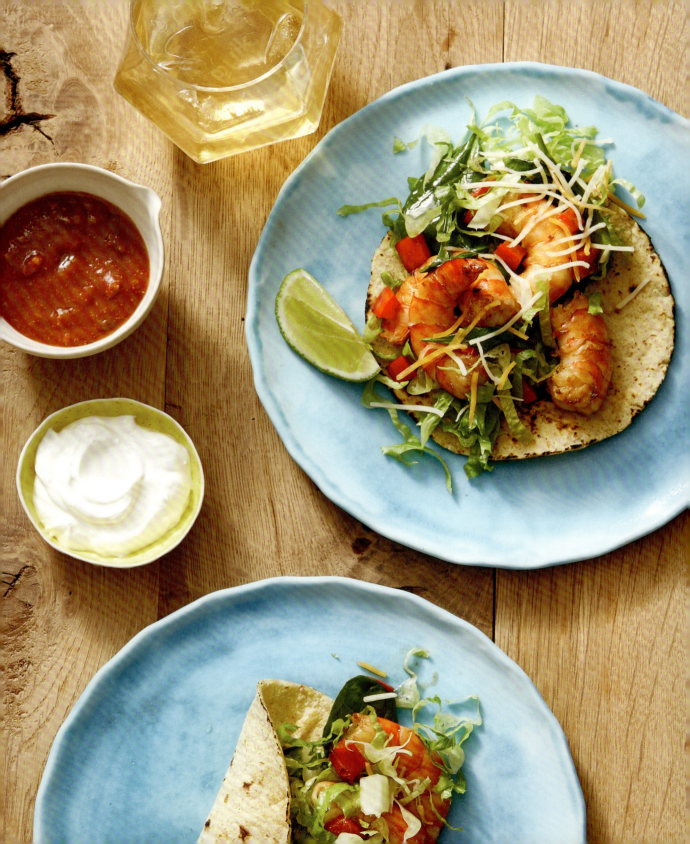

Shrimp Tacos with Sautéed Spinach

ACTIVE 10 MIN. | TOTAL 10 MIN. | SERVES 2

1 Heat a large skillet to medium-high and lightly coat with avocado oil spray.

2 Add shrimp and bell pepper. Cook about 2 minutes, flip, and cook for another 2 minutes until shrimp are pink. Remove and plate.

3 Meanwhile, in another large skillet on medium-high, heat avocado oil, salt and pepper, and spinach. Cook, stirring, for 5 minutes, or until desired tenderness.

4 Warm corn tortillas on a small skillet and cook until lightly browned, about 1 minute per side.

5 Top tortillas with cheese, then add shrimp and veggies to corn tortillas and top with taco sauce, chopped lettuce, and 2 Tbsp sour cream each.

NUTRITION (per serving): 350 cal, 32 g pro, 15 g carb, 6 g fiber, 1 g sugars (0 g added sugars), 19 g fat (8 g sat fat), 224 mg chol, 500 mg sodium

Avocado oil spray

½ lb shrimp

½ red bell pepper, thinly sliced

1 tsp avocado oil

1 dash of sea salt

Black pepper

8 cups baby spinach

2 medium whole-grain corn tortillas

1 oz shredded Mexican-style cheese

2 Tbsp low-FODMAP taco sauce (such as Fody brand)

½ cup chopped romaine lettuce

4 Tbsp sour cream

Chicken Margherita

1 In a large bowl, combine chicken, salt and pepper, olive oil, and Italian seasoning. Toss thoroughly.

2 Grill or broil chicken over medium-high heat for about 6 to 8 minutes on each side until cooked through. Top each piece of chicken with a slice of mozzarella cheese and cook another minute or so until melted.

3 Toss tomatoes, lemon juice, and basil together. Top each chicken breast with 2 Tbsp pesto, a scoop of tomatoes, and some freshly cracked black pepper. Serve immediately.

NUTRITION (per serving): 380 cal, 33 g pro, 5 g carb, 4 g fiber, 1 g sugars (0 g added sugars), 25 g fat (7 g sat fat), 106 mg chol, 242 mg sodium

2 4-oz boneless, skinless chicken breasts, pounded to less than 1-in. thickness

Salt and pepper, to taste

1 Tbsp olive oil

½ tsp Low-FODMAP Italian Seasoning (p. 102)

2 1-oz slices mozzarella cheese

½ cup cherry tomatoes, halved

½ Tbsp fresh lemon juice

⅛ cup packed basil leaves, very thinly sliced

¼ cup Low-FODMAP Pesto Sauce (p. 103)

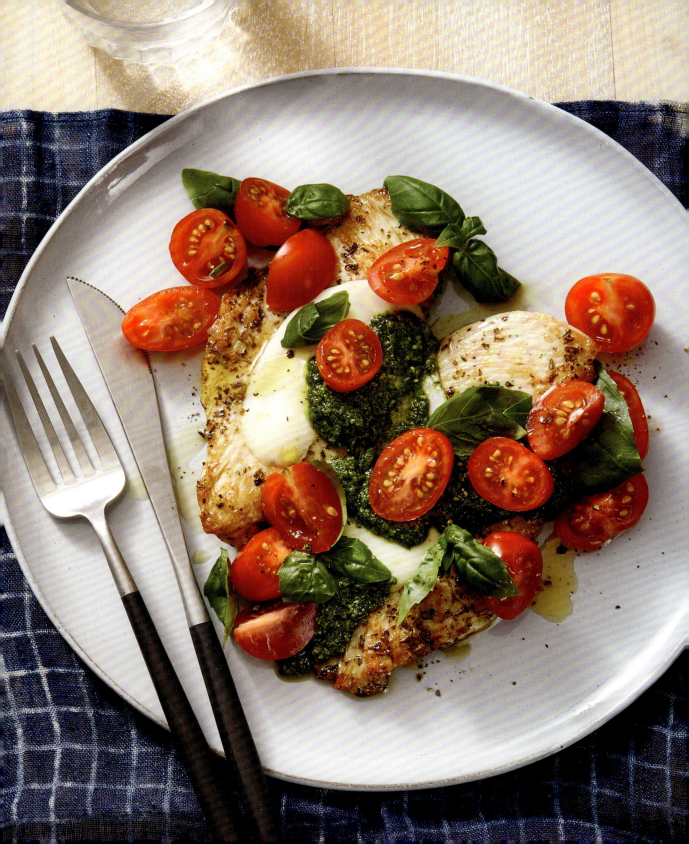

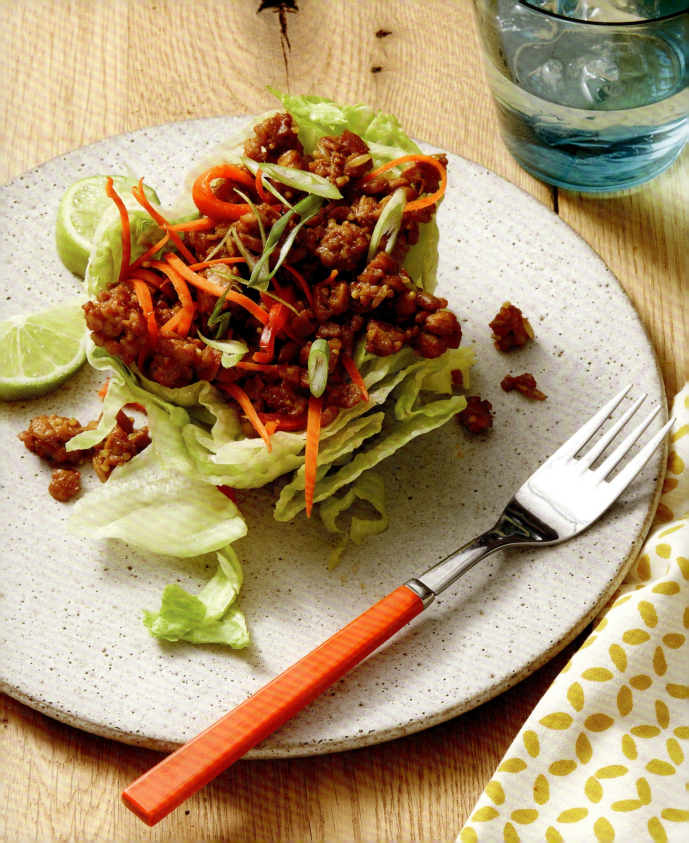

Tempeh in Lettuce Leaves

ACTIVE 20 MIN. | TOTAL 25 MIN. | SERVES 2

1 In a medium bowl, combine soy sauce, brown sugar, vinegar, sesame oil, and ginger.

2 Crumble the tempeh into small chunks and add to bowl.

3 In a large skillet over medium heat, warm olive oil. Add carrots and bell pepper. Cook until vegetables soften, 3 to 5 minutes.

4 Add tempeh mixture to skillet and stir. Cook until tempeh starts to brown, 5 minutes.

5 Stir in tapioca starch and cook, stirring continuously, until sauce thickens, 2 to 3 minutes. Add a small dash of salt and pepper to taste.

6 Spoon tempeh mixture into each lettuce cup. Top with sliced scallion tips and enjoy!

NUTRITION (per serving): 390 cal, 27 g pro, 25 g carb, 5 g fiber, 7 g sugars (7 g added sugars), 23 g fat (4.5 g sat fat), 0 mg chol, 880 mg sodium

¼ cup reduced-sodium soy sauce

1 Tbsp brown sugar, packed

1 Tbsp rice vinegar

1½ tsp sesame oil

¼ tsp finely sliced ginger

1 8-oz pkg. tempeh

1 Tbsp garlic-infused olive oil

1 carrot, thinly sliced

1 bell pepper, thinly sliced

1 Tbsp tapioca starch

½ head iceberg lettuce, washed and torn

Salt and pepper, to taste

1 scallion, thinly sliced (green parts only)

Taco Salad

1 In a large skillet over medium-high, heat the oil. Add turkey, breaking it up with a mixing spoon. Cook until lightly browned, about 5 minutes.

2 Add taco seasoning and water and simmer for approximately 8 minutes.

3 Split romaine into 2 bowls and add turkey meat. Top with beans, scallions, avocado, tomatoes, cheese, corn, sour cream, and lime juice. Add low-FODMAP salsa, if desired.

NUTRITION (per serving): 400 cal, 31 g pro, 21 g carb, 9 g fiber, 7.5 g sugars (0 g added sugars), 23 g fat (7.5 g sat fat), 100 mg chol, 280 mg sodium

2 tsp garlic-infused oil

1 lb ground turkey

1 Tbsp low-FODMAP taco seasoning (such as Fody brand)

½ cup water

8 cups romaine lettuce

¼ cup canned black beans, rinsed well

½ cup chopped scallions (green parts only)

¼ avocado, sliced

2 large beefsteak tomatoes, chopped

½ cup shredded Mexican-style cheese

¼ cup corn (frozen defrosted, fresh, or canned and rinsed)

2 Tbsp sour cream

1 Tbsp lime juice

Low-FODMAP salsa (p. 103)

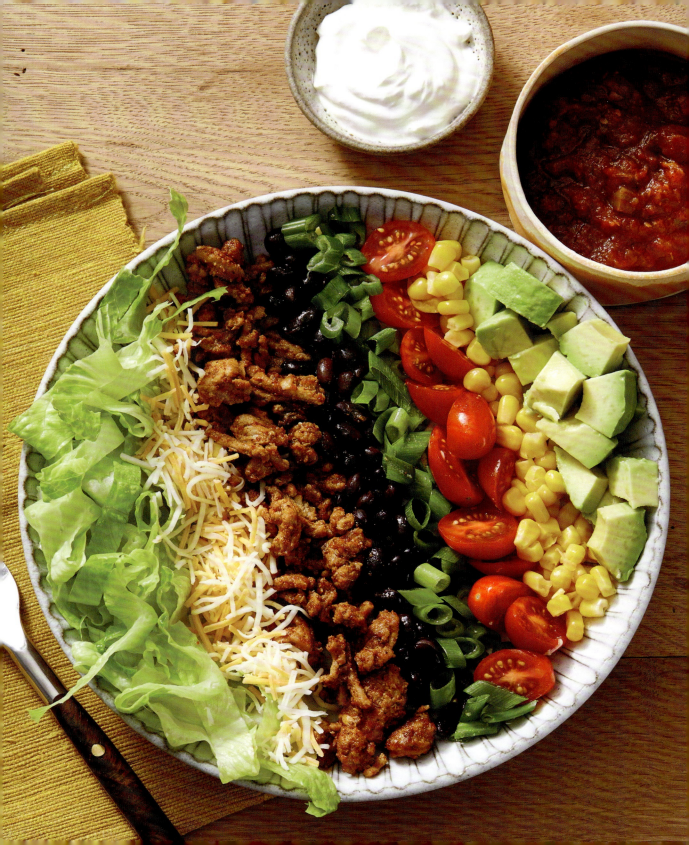

Low-FODMAP Condiments, Seasonings, and Extras

Low-FODMAP Marinara Sauce

ACTIVE 20 MIN. | TOTAL 20 MIN. | SERVES 8

1 In a blender, place all ingredients except salt. Pulse until desired sauce consistency is achieved.

2 In a large saucepan over medium-high heat, bring sauce to a boil. Reduce heat and let simmer for 15 minutes, stirring occasionally.

3 Season with salt and serve.

NUTRITION (per serving): 82 cal, 1 g pro, 5 g carb, 1.5 g fiber, 3.5 g sugars (0 g added sugars), 7 g fat (1 g sat fat), 0 mg chol, 480 mg sodium

1 28-oz can whole peeled tomatoes

¼ cup garlic-infused olive oil

½ tsp dried basil

¼ tsp dried oregano

⅛ tsp red pepper flakes, optional

Salt, to taste

Low-FODMAP Italian Seasoning

ACTIVE 5 MIN. | TOTAL 5 MIN. | SERVES 11

In a small bowl, mix all ingredients until well combined. Store in airtight container until ready to use.

1 Tbsp dried oregano

2 tsp dried thyme

2 tsp dried marjoram

1 tsp dried sage

1 tsp dried basil

1 tsp dried rosemary

⅛ tsp red pepper flakes

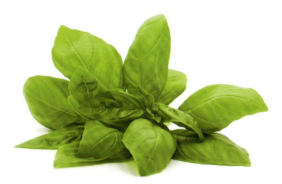

Low-FODMAP Pesto Sauce

ACTIVE 5 MIN. | TOTAL 5 MIN. | SERVES 8

In the bowl of a food processor, combine basil, pine nuts, scallions, and lemon juice. Process until roughly chopped. Slow processor to add oil. Season with sea salt.

NUTRITION (per serving): 106 cal, 1 g pro, 2 g carb, 1 g fiber, 0.5 g sugars (0 g added sugars), 11 g fat (2 g sat fat), 0 mg chol, 30 mg sodium

1½ oz fresh basil
(or 2 small pkgs.)

¼ cup pine nuts

¼ cup scallions
(green parts only)

Juice of ½ small lemon

¼ cup garlic-infused oil

Sea salt, to taste

Low-FODMAP Salsa

ACTIVE 5 MIN. | TOTAL 5 MIN. | SERVES 4

Mix all ingredients together for a fresh salsa!

NUTRITION (per serving): 15 cal, 1 g pro, 3.4 g carb, 1.5 g fiber, 1.5 g sugars (0 g added sugars), 0 g fat (0 g sat fat), 0 mg chol, 45 mg sodium

Tip: Refrigerate and save for up to 48 hours

6 medium vine-ripe or
beefsteak tomatoes,
chopped

¼ cup chopped scallions
(green parts only)

1 small cucumber,
chopped

2 Tbsp chopped fresh
cilantro leaves

2 tsp freshly squeezed lime
juice, more or less to taste

Kosher salt, to taste

Low-FODMAP Lemon Vinaigrette

ACTIVE 5 MIN. | TOTAL 5 MIN. | SERVES 6

¼ cup red wine vinegar

1 Tbsp Dijon mustard

½ tsp dried oregano

¼ tsp salt

½ cup garlic-infused olive oil

Juice of 1 lemon

Mix together all ingredients in a jar. Seal with lid and store for up to 1 week in the refrigerator.

Note: After storing in the fridge, olive oil may solidify. Let sit at room temperature for 30 minutes before serving to allow oil to liquify again.

NUTRITION (per 2 Tbsp): 180 cal, 0 g pro, 0 g carb, 0 g fiber, 0 g sugars (0 g added sugars), 18 g fat (1 g sat fat), 0 g chol, 129 mg sodium

Low-FODMAP Balsamic Vinaigrette

ACTIVE 5 MIN. | TOTAL 5 MIN. | SERVES 6

½ cup extra-virgin olive oil

¼ cup balsamic vinegar

2 tsp Dijon mustard

Salt and pepper, to taste

Mix together all ingredients in a jar. Seal with lid and store for up to 1 week in the refrigerator.

Note: After storing in the fridge, olive oil may solidify. Let sit at room temperature for 30 minutes before serving to allow oil to liquify again.

NUTRITION (per 2 Tbsp): 164 cal, 0 g pro, 1 g carb, 0 g fiber, 1 g sugars (0 g added sugars), 17 g fat (2 g sat fat), 0 g chol, 68 mg sodium

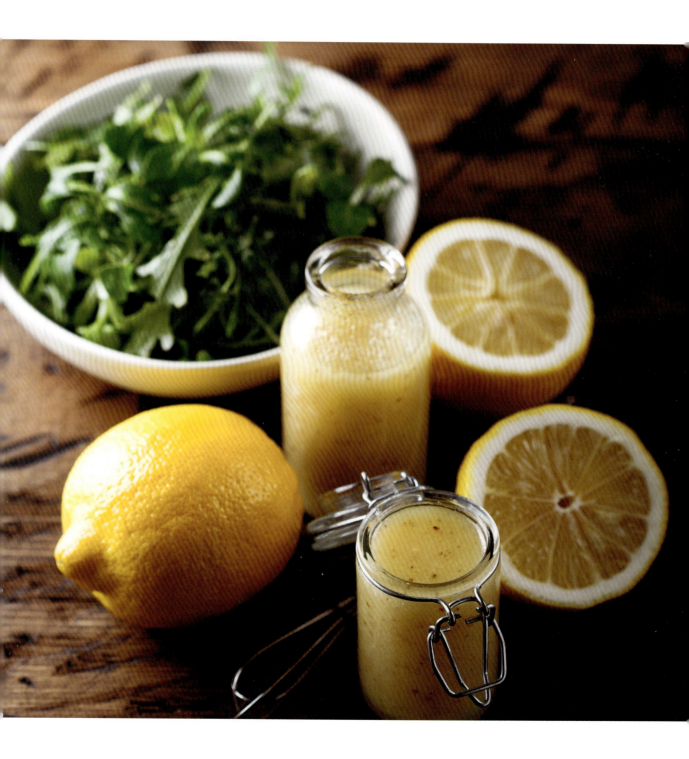

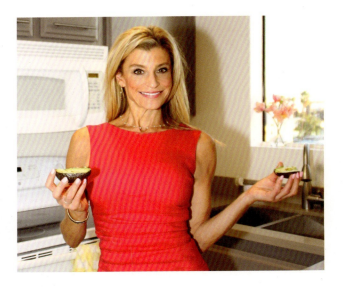

About the Expert

Sarah Mirkin R.D.N., is a registered dietitian and owner of the private practice Kitchen Coach in Beverly Hills, CA. Sarah works with people all over the world online and via telephone or video chat to help them overcome obstacles and reach their health and wellness goals permanently. She has been practicing for 23 years. Follow her low-FODMAP journey on Instagram @kitchencoachRD or schedule an online session with Sarah by visiting kitchencoachrd.com.